Stretching For Dummies®

Stretches to Start Your Day With

If you want to start your day out right, keep this handy list of stretches on your nightstand so you can practice them first thing in the morning.

- ✔ **Knees to chest:** Bring both knees toward your chest, placing one hand under each knee for support. Breathe deeply and hold the stretch for 30 seconds. (See Chapter 9.)

- ✔ **Total body stretch:** Lie on your back with your arms extended over your head. Inhale deeply and stretch your arms and legs as far as you can in opposite directions. As you exhale, release the stretch and relax your whole body. Repeat this exercise three or four times, each time trying to reach and stretch a little farther. (See Chapter 9.)

- ✔ **Spinal rotation:** Lie on your back with your knees bent and place a pillow next to you. Bring both knees toward your chest, placing your hands under each knee for support. Take a deep breath in, and as you exhale, slowly lower your legs to one side until they rest on the pillow. Try to keep your opposite shoulder blade and your head on the bed or a pillow, so you're just hinging at the hips. Hold this stretch for about 30 seconds, taking several deep breaths as you relax into the stretch. (See Chapter 9.)

Stuck-in-Traffic or Sitting-at-Your-Desk Stretches

If you sit all day or commute to work (who doesn't do one of those things?!), here are a few stretches to help you work out the kinks:

- ✔ **Shoulder and neck stretch:** Sit tall in your chair with your feet flat on the floor, your abdominals lifted, and your hands resting on your thighs. Slowly rotate your shoulders forward, up, back, and down as if you were drawing a circle with your shoulders. Breathe deeply as you repeat this motion four to six times. (See Chapter 10.)

- ✔ **Seated chest stretch:** Sit tall with both your feet flat on the floor and your back flat against the back of your chair. Clasp your hands together behind your head. Inhale, and as you exhale, gently press your elbows back, squeeze your shoulder blades together, and lift your chin and chest toward the ceiling. Hold the stretch for about 30 seconds, and then release back to starting position. (See Chapter 10.)

- ✔ **Wrist and forearm stretch:** Sit up straight in your chair with the palm of one hand pressing against the fingers of the other hand. Point your fingers upward and keep your elbows lifting toward the ceiling. Inhale, and as you exhale, gently press the heel of your hand against your fingers. Hold this stretch for 30 seconds and repeat on the other side. (See Chapter 10.)

Remedies for Sore Muscles

The next time you're in pain, there are a few things you can do to speed your recovery along. The following list gives you a few suggestions for helping your sore muscles get back to feeling good again:

- ✔ Apply an ice pack for 20 minutes to any area that is sore. Repeat this every hour until the pain subsides.

- ✔ Stretch the sore area gently to help your body get rid of lactic acid, which helps contribute to the pain.

- ✔ Be sure to walk 10 to 20 minutes at least once a day to increase circulation throughout your body. This helps deliver much-needed oxygen to your sore muscles.

- ✔ Drink at least eight glasses of water daily to stay hydrated and help flush out the lactic acid in your sore muscles.

- ✔ Avoid any strenuous activity as long as you're in pain.

For Dummies: Bestselling Book Series for Beginners

Stretching For Dummies®

Top Five Anywhere, Anytime Stretches

The following five stretches are my personal all-time favorites — they're fun, easy to do, and amazingly effective!

- **Neck stretch:** Find a sturdy chair that you can sit comfortably in and lightly grasp the base of the chair with your right hand. Slowly rotate your head to the left as you lean forward slightly. Hold this position, maintaining the light to medium stretch for at least one full minute. Repeat on the other side by simply reversing the instructions. (See Chapter 4.)

- **Chest stretch:** Kneel on a carpeted floor or mat with your forearms crossed and resting on the seat of a sturdy chair. Inhale, and as you exhale, let your head and chest sink below the chair. Hold the stretch for 30 seconds, breathing deeply to help you sink gradually deeper into the stretch. (See Chapter 4.)

- **Supported upper back stretch:** Stand with your feet hip-width apart and place your hands on a sturdy surface for support. Walk your feet back far enough that you can extend your arms as you move your chest toward the floor. Exhale and press your chest toward the floor and your hips toward the ceiling so you have a slight arch in your back. Hold the stretch for 20 to 30 seconds. (See Chapter 4.)

- **Standing quad stretch:** Stand up tall and place your right hand on a stable surface. Inhale and lift your left knee toward the sky and grab hold of your left ankle (or top of your foot) with your left hand. Exhale and slowly lower your left knee, gently moving your left foot toward your left buttocks. To really feel this stretch correctly, try to tuck your pelvis under, thinking about your tailbone moving toward the floor. Hold this stretch for 30 seconds and repeat with the right leg. (See Chapter 7.)

- **Standing calf stretch:** Face a wall or sturdy surface and stand one foot away with your feet together. Lean forward, place your hands on the wall in front of you, and move your right foot back as far as you can with your heel on the floor. Bend your left knee slightly, keeping your right knee straight. Take a deep breath in, and as you exhale, gently press your hips forward, keeping your right heel on the ground. Hold the stretch for several deep breaths, and then slightly bend your right knee without lifting your heel off the floor. Repeat with your left leg. (See Chapter 7.)

My Favorite Stretches to Alleviate Back Pain

Here they are! My favorite stretches to help ease back pain and just make you feel better in general:

- **Standing pelvic tilts:** Place your back against a wall and bend your knees so that you're in a slight squat. Rest your hands on your thighs just above your knees. Take a deep breath in, and as you exhale, slowly tilt your pelvis forward until you feel your lower back against the wall. Inhale and release the stretch by moving your pelvis back to the starting position. Exhale and tilt your pelvis again. (See Chapter 6.)

- **Alternating knees to chest:** Lie on your back with your knees bent and your feet flat on the floor. Inhale deeply, and as you exhale, bring your right knee up toward your chest, placing your hands behind the knee for guidance and assistance. Hold the stretch for 30 seconds, and then lower your leg back to the beginning position and repeat the stretch with your left leg. (See Chapter 6.)

- **Kneeling pelvic tilt:** Get on your hands and knees, making sure to keep your back relaxed and not arched. Inhale, and as you exhale, pull your butt forward, rotating the pubic bone upward. Hold this position for three seconds and then relax. (See Chapter 13.)

- **Seated upper back stretch:** Sit on the floor with your knees slightly bent and your arms crossed behind your knees. Inhale as you lean forward, letting your chest rest on your thighs. As you exhale, round your back and pull away from your knees, but be sure that your arms are locked under your knees. Hold this position for 20 to 30 seconds. (See Chapter 4.)

For Dummies: Bestselling Book Series for Beginners

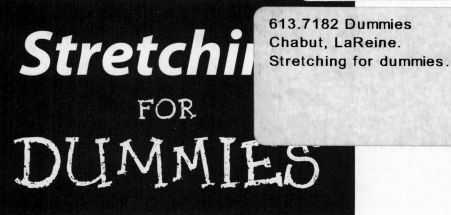

Stretching FOR DUMMIES

by LaReine Chabut

with Madeleine Lewis

BICENTENNIAL
1807
WILEY
2007
BICENTENNIAL

Wiley Publishing, Inc.

Stretching For Dummies®

Published by
Wiley Publishing, Inc.
111 River St.
Hoboken, NJ 07030-5774
www.wiley.com

For general information on our other products and services, please contact our Customer Care Department within the U.S. at 800-762-2974, outside the U.S. at 317-572-3993, or fax 317-572-4002.

For technical support, please visit www.wiley.com/techsupport.

Wiley also publishes its books in a variety of electronic formats. Some content that appears in print may not be available in electronic books.

Library of Congress Control Number: 2006939586

ISBN: 978-0-470-06741-3

Manufactured in the United States of America

10 9 8 7 6 5 4 3 2

WILEY

About the Author

LaReine Chabut is a lifestyle and fitness expert, model, and mom. She's the author of *Exercise Balls For Dummies* (Wiley) and *Lose That Baby Fat!* (M. Evans) and is a contributing fitness expert for *Shape Fit Pregnancy* magazine. LaReine has served as the lead instructor for America's number one exercise video series *The Firm* (over three million copies sold worldwide) and has graced the covers of such high-profile fitness publications as *Shape, Health, New Body,* and *Runner's World.* She has appeared on CNN, ABC, FOX News, EXTRA, Access Hollywood, Good Day LA, and KABC and is a premier trainer for Ipods (see www.podfitness.com/lareinechabut) along with Kathy Smith, David Kirsch, and other top trainers in their field.

As an actress, LaReine penned a sitcom with Meg Ryan entitled *Below the Radar* for the Fox Network and Castle Rock Entertainment. She has co-written and starred in two short films: *Separation Anxiety,* which broadcast on Lifetime Television, and *Good Jill Hunting,* which aired on the Sundance Channel. Her series regular and guest starring appearances include *Linc's, Nash Bridges, The Secret World of Alex Mack, USA High, The Single Guy, Strange Luck, Murder She Wrote,* and *Quantum Leap,* to name a handful.

To read more about LaReine, check out her Web sites at www.lareinechabut.com or www.losethatbabyfat.com.

Dedication

To my newborn daughter Sofia Rose (who arrived on the first deadline of this book), her new big sister Bella, and my husband Bobby . . . you are my world. And to the many readers who purchase this book because they need a good stretch — I hope you get one!

Author's Acknowledgments

Stretching For Dummies is my third book, and once again I have to thank Rob Dyer at Wiley for encouraging me to write in the first place. I certainly couldn't have done it without his guidance. My literary agent, Danielle Egan-Miller, also deserves big thanks for pushing me to write this book, knowing that the birth of my second daughter was on the horizon (she's a mom, too, and knows how hard it is to multitask). That being said, I have to give special thanks to Madeleine Lewis for all her help . . . I couldn't have done it without her.

Writing a book such as this requires a lot of teamwork, so I'd like to thank the entire staff at Wiley, including Kristin DeMint, my project editor, who was very enthusiastic with the material and really made the book flow. Lindsay Lefevere, acquisitions editor, who couldn't believe there wasn't a *For Dummies* book on stretching and called me on Stacy Kennedy's suggestion. Copy editor, Carrie Burchfield, for making my sentences flow smoothly, and photo editor Carmen Krikorian, who once again helped me produce such fantastic photos. The photographer, Tilden Patterson (who also had a new baby a few weeks after me), deserves a big thanks for making everybody look so good and for shooting 165 stretches in one day! You're awesome, Tilden . . . And special thanks from Madeleine Lewis to Dr. Jerry Hizon MD, FAAFP, and to Denise Klatte, MPT, for sharing their knowledge and perspective.

Publisher's Acknowledgments

We're proud of this book; please send us your comments through our Dummies online registration form located at www.dummies.com/register/.

Some of the people who helped bring this book to market include the following:

Acquisitions, Editorial, and Media Development

Project Editor: Kristin DeMint

Acquisitions Editor: Lindsay Lefevere

Copy Editor: Carrie A. Burchfield

Technical Editor: David L. Walston, ATC; Assistant Athletic Trainer for the Indianapolis Colts

Senior Editorial Manager: Jennifer Ehrlich

Editorial Assistants: Erin Calligan, Joe Niesen, David Lutton, Leeann Harney

Cover Photos: © Tilden Patterson (www.tildenphoto.com)

Cartoons: Rich Tennant (www.the5thwave.com)

Composition Services

Project Coordinator: Jennifer Theriot

Layout and Graphics: Melanee Prendergast, Heather Ryan

Anniversary Logo Design: Richard Pacifico

Proofreaders: John Greenough, Jessica Kramer, Susan Moritz, Techbooks

Indexer: Techbooks

Special Help
Carmen Krikorian

Publishing and Editorial for Consumer Dummies

Diane Graves Steele, Vice President and Publisher, Consumer Dummies

Joyce Pepple, Acquisitions Director, Consumer Dummies

Kristin A. Cocks, Product Development Director, Consumer Dummies

Michael Spring, Vice President and Publisher, Travel

Kelly Regan, Editorial Director, Travel

Publishing for Technology Dummies

Andy Cummings, Vice President and Publisher, Dummies Technology/General User

Composition Services

Gerry Fahey, Vice President of Production Services

Debbie Stailey, Director of Composition Services

Contents at a Glance

Exercises at a Glance

Lower-Body Stretches

Morning, Midday, and Evening Stretches

Stretches for Working and Traveling

Warm-Up and Cool-Down Stretches

Sports-Specific Stretches

Pregnacy-Friendly Stretches

Kid-Friendly Stretches

Senior-Friendly Stretches

Back and Shoulders Stretch

Table of Contents

Introduction

●●●

Stretching is a hot topic these days — just take a look when you attend any sporting event and you can see multitudes of athletes doing side bends or stretching out their calves or some other body part. Yes, stretching is good for your body, plus it helps prevent injuries and manage day-to-day stress!

But what is stretching? Well, it really is best described as any movement that increases your range of motion and tests your individual flexibility. So for example, stretching can be as easy as turning your head from side to side or just touching your toes. In fact, some people call stretching flexibility training because you do just that — train your muscles to be more flexible through the use of simple movements.

Just think of all the little ways in your daily life that flexibility comes in handy: backing your car out of the driveway or reaching for something on the top shelf or bending over to tie your shoe! For those reasons (and many more), stretching keeps your muscles long and pliable and enhances your life to keep your movements pain free forever (or as long as possible).

About This Book

This book introduces you to various stretch exercises for everyone — no matter what your age or lifestyle. The chapters in this book can help you develop a regular, everyday stretch routine or just discover a few new moves to keep you feeling great! The stretches consist of yoga stretches, children stretches, sports stretches, and more. You also discover how to prevent workout boredom by adding a few new props, such as a foam roller, a strap, a block, or my personal favorite, the exercise ball. In addition, I cover simple stretches you can do at work and on the go or even when you're simply sitting around.

This book also contains comprehensive stretching sections for special circumstances: pregnancy, lower back pain, and even aches and pains. Whatever your interest or age, you're sure to get a good stretch and have some fun doing it! Here's a sampling of some of the questions that you can find answers to:

- ✔ How long should I hold a stretch?
- ✔ What muscles am I using when I stretch a particular body part?
- ✔ Are you supposed to wear shoes when you stretch?
- ✔ What kind of changes can I expect to see in my body from stretching?
- ✔ How many days a week should I stretch?
- ✔ Is it safe to stretch during pregnancy?
- ✔ What are the best stretch exercises I can do for back pain?
- ✔ Can kids stretch too?
- ✔ Can I stretch out my core?
- ✔ Is it safe for senior citizens to stretch?
- ✔ Are there stretches I can do for menstrual cramps?
- ✔ Will the stretches be challenging enough for me if I'm already in shape?
- ✔ Are there stretches that can help relieve headaches?

Conventions Used in This Book

This book focuses on stretching in different situations while emphasizing safety and proper body alignment. Make sure to read the step-by-step instructions located next to the photo illustrations *before* you try out any of the stretches. By following that guideline, your stretches will be easier and safer.

Also keep in mind that most of the stretch illustrations are shown in two stages, labeled with the figure number and also with *a* and *b,* which demonstrate the beginning and end of poses.

Here are a few additional conventions:

- ✔ I use *italics* to point out any new terms or bits of jargon you should know.
- ✔ Web sites and e-mail addresses appear in `monofont` to help them stand out.
- ✔ The numbered sets of instructions for the stretches and the keywords in lists appear in **boldface.**

What You're Not to Read

Although I feel that all the information in this book is important, the sidebars that appear in the gray boxes don't contain information that you absolutely need to know in order to get a good stretch. However, these sidebars do contain great tips and information about your health, so I encourage you to read them at some point.

Foolish Assumptions

This book, like all *For Dummies* books, has a friendly and approachable tone that assumes you don't know a whole lot about stretching — not that you're an actual dummy! I also make a few other assumptions about you, the reader:

- ✔ You're interested in stretching and want to make it part of your daily life.
- ✔ You don't have much experience with stretching.
- ✔ You're ready, willing, and able to find out more about stretching and how to do the stretches in this book.

If this sounds like you, then you've come to the right place!

How This Book Is Organized

Stretching For Dummies is divided into five different parts, each one with a unique focus. You can go directly to whichever part interests you the most or start at the beginning of the book to gather some information and a checklist of what you need to know before beginning each stretching chapter. In the following sections, I outline the different parts and what you can find in them.

Part I: The Why's, Where's, When's, and How's of Letting Loose and Snapping Back

If you're new to stretching, Part I is a great section for you to read first. Part I covers all the important issues you want (and need) to know *before* you begin your stretch program:

- ✔ Who should stretch?
- ✔ How often you should stretch?
- ✔ What test stretches help you find your own individual flexibility?
- ✔ What props you can use when you stretch?
- ✔ What are the benefits of stretching?

In Part I, I also offer a worksheet (in Chapter 3) to help you determine your flexibility and chart your progress as you move through your stretching program.

Part II: Head, Shoulders, Knees, and Toes: Targeting Specific Areas

Part II is organized in a very logical manner — Chapter 4 starts off with a series of upper body stretches, and then the chapters progress with stretch series that are illustrated for various individual body parts. Finally, Chapter 8 finishes with a total body workout to stretch your entire body.

Because I believe you should work out in a progressive manner (either from the top of the body moving downward or from the bottom of the body and working upward), I strongly encourage starting with the upper body in Chapter 4 and progressing through the chapters until you reach Chapter 8. These chapters concentrate first on the upper body, the core, the lower back, and finally your lower body.

Part III: From the Daily Grind to Ways to Unwind: Routines to Fit Your Life and Needs

Part III shows you a variety of stretches that you can adapt to your individual lifestyle. This part of the book may be the most useful part if you have an issue with stretching during the workday or if you have a particular sport you do and want to add a few new moves.

In Chapter 9, I tell you how to stretch in bed before getting up in the morning and offer you a few stretches you can do before turning in for the night. These stretches really get your day going and then help you wind down and get a good night's sleep. Chapter 11 contains a basic warm-up and cool-down routine that can be added to any workout or used alone. You also find a few stretches for tension headaches in Chapter 10. Chapter 12 contains stretches for various sports that you may be involved in.

Part IV: Getting Limber As You Live: Stretches for Various Life Stages

Part IV is a fantastic section that focuses on stretching during the special circumstances in your life. If you're pregnant, check out Chapter 13. This chapter contains photo illustrations of stretches and strengthening exercises that help prepare you for that big day.

Chapter 14 is a fun-filled chapter for stretching for kids. Whether your little ones are 4 years old (like my daughter Bella in the photos) or 14, they can do these simple and easy movements at home with their friends or brothers and sisters.

The last chapter of Part IV is Chapter 15. The chapter focuses on stretching for seniors. The exercises are both fun and practical and should keep you strong and flexible for years to come.

Part V: The Part of Tens

In every *For Dummies* book, you find The Part of Tens. Part V contains two chapters of top-ten lists of fun facts about the different ways you can stretch and what you can use to enhance your workout. Chapter 16 lists ten common aches and pains and tells you how stretching can help get rid of them. And in Chapter 17, I offer ten things you can find around the house to use as stretching accessories. Can you believe a fireplace tool is one of them?

Icons Used in This Book

As you flip through this book, you see a lot of different graphics in the margins. Those pics are called *icons,* and they give you useful information along the way. Reading the info in these icons before you try the actual stretches is helpful because many of them suggest easier or better ways of performing each one.

Here's a list of icons used in this book:

The tip icon gives you useful information that (hopefully) makes your life easier as it relates to stretching and flexibility. I may point you to a specific chapter or resource or provide hints to modify an exercise to change the level of difficulty.

As you may have guessed, this icon points out really important information that you need to keep in mind. Very valuable information comes with these icons, so don't skip 'em!

The warning icon highlights information that keeps you from hurting yourself. You should read the information next to this icon *before* you attempt each stretch. You'll be glad you did!

Where to Go from Here

Stretching For Dummies is a reference guide for beginners and an introduction to performing stretches. You can start reading at the very beginning of this book to gather a little information first, or you can dive right in and tear out the yellow Cheat Sheet in the front of this book to take it with you as you're running out the door to a stretch class.

If you're not sure where you want to start, I suggest browsing through the table of contents to get a sense of exactly what this book covers and what topics interest you. You may find that you already know the basics but have always wanted to know how to use a stretching strap, so you can immediately flip to that chapter (which is Chapter 3).

If you fall into one of the special circumstances groups, you may want to go directly to that section to find which chapter covers your special needs. (Part IV is the section in question.) If you're like me, you may just want to go directly to the workout chapters that pertain to you to figure out some new moves.

And if you already know a lot about stretching and just want to brush up on your technique a bit, you can turn to the index to find out which information pertains to you. No matter where you choose to start, it's great that you're here. Enjoy the journey to your new body!

Part I

The Why's, Where's, When's, and How's of Letting Loose and Snapping Back

The 5th Wave · By Rich Tennant

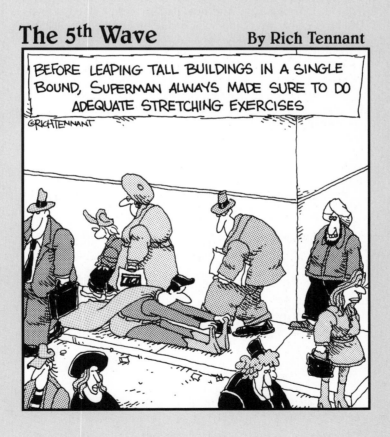

BEFORE LEAPING TALL BUILDINGS IN A SINGLE BOUND, SUPERMAN ALWAYS MADE SURE TO DO ADEQUATE STRETCHING EXERCISES

In this part . . .

1 know that you know stretching is good for you, but in Chapter 1, I cover *why* stretching is so good for you, and I answer all your stretching questions: When do I stretch? Why should I stretch? And how do I stretch? I also get into the science of stretching, which can lend some insight into what's happening inside your muscles as they stretch.

Chapter 2 includes everything you need to know to get started stretching, including what props you might want to use and how much space you need. I also give you the basics of a safe stretching program, including exactly how each stretch should feel.

And finally, in Chapter 3, I show you how to test your present level of flexibility, so you can figure out your starting point for your new stretching program. I even help you understand what flexibility is and talk about what you can change (and what you can't).

Chapter 1

Here a Stretch, There a Stretch, Everywhere a Stretch, Stretch

Stretching is a powerful tool that you can always have access to and only requires a few simple movements (kind of like having your own ruby slippers). And the results can certainly be just like magic: new ease of movement, an increase in your physical capabilities, and deep composure that requires you to do nothing more than breathe.

Many of you may have been taught to fear and dread stretching by overbearing PE teachers who forced you to touch your toes. But the ideas and techniques I describe in this book were never heard in your parents' PE class (or mine for that matter). This training is a kinder, gentler form of flexibility based on hard science and decades of practical experience. And the key insight is that stretching is *not* supposed to hurt!

If this book has one mission, it's to demonstrate that stretching is easy and simple, or in other words, stretching is your friend. All the amazing benefits of stretching can be yours anywhere, anytime, without spending a dime (other than buying this book, of course). And it's really just as easy as clicking your heels like Dorothy in *The Wizard of Oz!*

The Why's of Stretching

Go ahead — ask your doctor, your trainer, your physical therapist, or your chiropractor whether you should stretch. Get ready to hear the exact same answer from all of them: a resounding *yes*. Even though they don't make a dime giving such advice, why would all these professionals so enthusiastically recommend stretching? The long list of amazing answers follows in this section.

You stand taller, look thinner, and your body works its best

Correct posture not only makes you look taller and thinner, but also it allows your body to perform the way it was meant to. What's more, good posture aids dramatically in facilitating free and effective breathing.

The main enemy of good posture however is tight muscles! Stretching can help you correct muscular imbalances that lead to incorrect skeletal alignment. One cause of this kind of imbalance is using one side of your body more than the other. Times that you may do this include

- ✔ Carrying your toddler on the same side of your body
- ✔ Carrying your briefcase in the same hand everyday
- ✔ Wearing your shoulder bag on the same shoulder
- ✔ Sleeping on the same side
- ✔ Using the same shoulder to cradle the phone while you're talking
- ✔ Using the same arm to put around your sweetie on a date

Such chronic imbalances can rob you of energy and efficiency in movement, or even result in back pain. So switch it up, and stretch regularly to help balance out these bad habits. Also be sure to stand up straight!

You can twist farther and feel looser

Over time, muscles naturally tend to shorten and become tight. So as you age, your ability to fully utilize movement in your body becomes compromised. Think about it: If a muscle is already in a chronically shortened state, then it can never attain its full power potential when you try to contract it because it's already semicontracted. A tight muscle limits your range of motion, and you can easily hurt yourself.

A few words to live by: Don't eat seafood in a month without an "R" in it, let sleeping dogs lie, and a tight muscle is a weak muscle. Ignore any of these time-tested maxims at your peril, and chances are, one way or another, you're going to get bitten.

Stretching increases your ability to function daily — called *functional flexibility.* This flexibility helps dramatically increase the range of motion in your joints, which enhances your performance in your chosen sport and helps in your everyday life by making it possible for you to reach higher or lower, bend farther, and reduce nagging aches and pains from tight, tense muscles.

Lack of functional flexibility can make small everyday movements annoying and even painful.

You help nip injuries in the bud

Numerous studies claim that stretching exercises increase flexibility and decrease the severity of injuries and the time it takes to recover from an injury. Stretching can actually reduce the chance of being injured in the first place, too!

Stretching reduces muscle sprain or joint strain in case of accidental overstretching of muscles or joints when engaging in sports or other physical activities. In short, although nothing can prevent injury completely, stretching can be a very low-cost, long-term insurance policy for your body — whether you engage in sports or not.

You keep stress from getting the best of you

Stress is a part of life! Some stress (even a little) is good because it can spur you on to take action and achieve great things. But too much stress can actually threaten your health and well being, resulting in depression, anxiety, and memory loss.

Stretching can be therapeutic for many people as *one* way to relieve stress. (You may already have an entire arsenal of things you do to relieve stress.) Of course, stretching can help individual muscles release and relax, but the deep, regular breathing that's so important to effective stretching can also oxygenate your blood and reduce overall stress and anxiety. What's more, the slow, meticulous movements in a good flexibility program can provide a meditative effect. And focusing intensely on the muscles you're stretching can help clear your mind of distractions. In the end, stretching can help make you more flexible, inside and out.

You keep your muscles from feeling achy

Current research suggests that stretching can reduce that post-exercise tight, tender feeling called *delayed onset muscle soreness* (DOMS). For decades many people thought this achy feeling was the result of lactic acid buildup in the tissues of your muscles. But it turns out they were wrong because lactic acid is a normal byproduct, resulting from the chemical reaction of muscle contraction during exercise.

So now cutting-edge thinking attributes this discomfort to tiny tears in muscle fibers caused by the requirements of unfamiliar training (also known as *eccentric* movements). By ensuring that your muscles are elastic and you have full range of motion in your joints, stretching protects you from sustaining the microscopic injuries caused by newly intense levels of exercise.

Stretching also decreases tension in your muscles and joints. Persistent muscle tightness can take a toll on your body by choking off blood flow to the muscles, which can result in raised blood pressure. This tightness can also decrease oxygen and nutrients in the muscle tissues, which in turn can cause the buildup of toxic waste products in the cells. The end result is persistent fatigue, as well as aches and pains in your tense muscles.

What's more, if a muscle stays partially contracted for an abnormally long time, the muscle can actually begin to shorten, which decreases range of motion and weakens the muscle, creating tightness and making the muscle less effective. A perpetually contracted muscle requires more energy to move than a relaxed muscle, so you wind up wasting energy with every movement.

So start a regular stretching program today to help reduce tension and tenderness in your muscles; the exercise can actually elevate the level of your overall health. Pretty amazing just from bending over and touching your toes!

The FAQs When It Comes to Stretching

Who, what, where, when, and why should you stretch? These questions are a few of the ones that you find answers to in the following sections.

When should 1 stretch?

Many trainers tell you to stretch either first thing in the morning or at the end of the day — or both. However, the rule of thumb is that you may stretch any time as long as your muscles are first warmed up (which means you've done at least five minutes of walking, hiking, biking, swimming, or calisthenics such as jumping jacks). Warming up your body properly allows you to gradually increase your circulation and get your blood flowing, which in turn makes you more flexible.

Picking a time that's just right for you, on the other hand, is an entirely different problem. And trying to force yourself into a schedule that doesn't really work certainly won't help you to stick with any flexibility program. So it's best to find a time of day that's most convenient for you and make that your special time for stretching . . . your body will thank you for the regular routine, and you'll soon see results.

How often should 1 stretch a particular muscle?

To increase flexibility in a muscle, generally you should stretch that muscle at least once a day. Elite athletes stretch even more than that — two to three times a day. But being realistic, the majority of people aren't professional athletes (and aren't getting *paid* the big bucks to stay stretched and fit), so finding the time to stretch that much can be difficult.

If you want to increase your present level of flexibility, engage in a focused flexibility program every other day to give your body a chance to rest and rejuvenate in between sessions. And when this pace of stretching becomes comfortable for you, maintain your new range of motion by stretching four to five times a week.

How long should 1 hold each stretch?

Studies demonstrate that the optimum effectiveness of a stretching exercise is reached after holding that stretch for approximately 30 seconds. If you stretch less, you don't really give your muscles time to fully lengthen and adapt to the exercise; stretching longer hasn't been proven to provide any additional benefits either. So stick with the 30-second rule, which equates to four to five slow, deep breaths.

For the scientist in you

If the doctor or scientist inside you is dying to know how the muscles technically work, here's the breakdown on the way your body makes the majority of its movements:

- A primary muscle (the *agonist*) is assisted by one or more secondary muscles (the *synergists*);

- Together they stretch the opposing muscle (the *antagonist*).

For example, when you bend your knee, the muscles on the back of your leg, including your hamstring (the agonist) and your gastrocnemius (your calf — the synergist) contract, which in turn stretches the quadriceps (the antagonist). Another example would be during a biceps curl: The biceps is the agonist, and the triceps is the antagonist . . . Got it?

How intense should the stretch be?

A stretch should feel no more than slightly uncomfortable. When you reach the point of resistance in your muscle, hold that stretch. In a few more days of stretching that muscle, you'll be able to comfortably move past that point.

When it comes to stretching, the old cliché "no pain, no gain" is dead wrong. In fact, pain is the most precise indicator of a stretch that has gone too far, either in degree or in duration. If you're stretching to the point where your muscle sizzles inside, or is quivering, or you actually find that you're becoming less flexible, back off. If you force a stretch, the strain can only set you back further than you were when you started.

Should I see a doctor before I begin a stretching program?

You should always consult a physician before embarking on any new fitness program — even a seemingly low-impact program such as stretching. And speaking to your healthcare professional is crucial before undertaking a regular flexibility program if you have arthritis, osteoporosis, or an injury that hasn't healed completely.

Try the stretches in Chapter 16, which are specifically for common aches and pains. And your doctor can advise you about specific stretches to focus on or to avoid and can help customize a stretching program to help meet your unique needs.

Should I stretch my muscles in a particular sequence?

After stretching a particular muscle group, you want to move on to a completely different muscle group so you don't overly fatigue that one group. The following list is my suggestion of the order in which to stretch your muscles:

1. Back (see Chapters 4 and 6)

2. Sides (see Chapters 5 and 8)

3. Neck (see Chapters 4 and 8)

4. Forearm and wrists (see Chapters 4, 8, 10, and 12)

5. Triceps (see Chapters 4, 8, and 12)

6. Chest (see Chapters 4, 8, 10, and 12)

7. Buttocks (see Chapters 5–8)

8. Groin (see Chapters 7, 8, 11, and 12)

9. Thighs (see Chapters 7, 8, 11, and 12)

10. Calves (see Chapters 7–12)

11. Shins (see Chapters 7–12)

12. Hamstrings (see Chapters 7–12)

Of course you can stretch one, some, or a handful of these areas, and if you stretch slowly and with control, you still receive all the benefits stretching has to offer. The model of the steps above is just one (really good) example of a progressive, complementary, full-body routine.

Differentiating between Two Types of Stretches

Stretching always bears the same concepts: to lengthen muscles and improve the range of motion in joints. But just like ice cream, stretching comes in different flavors. The two main categories of stretching techniques are dynamic stretches and static stretches. *Dynamic stretches* involve movement, whereas *static stretches* are held steadily. Because both of these techniques have different benefits and advantages, I cover both in this book.

Static stretches

Static stretching involves stretching to the farthest point you comfortably can and then holding the stretch (usually for 30 seconds). This technique is used primarily throughout this book for two reasons:

- ✔ They're the simplest and easiest form of stretching to master and perform correctly, so they're excellent for anyone new to flexibility training.
- ✔ The simplicity of the movements and the slow and gentle pace allow for mindful relaxation of the entire body.

Holding a comfortable position for 30 seconds or so allows your muscles to actually become accustomed to being stretched, which reduces your *stretch reflex* — a natural mechanism whereby a muscle under stress automatically contracts to protect itself. A gentle static stretch overcomes this natural defense mechanism and allows your muscles to efficiently relax and let go.

In the interests of full disclosure, static stretching can be further divided into two different types: static-passive and static-active.

- ✔ *Static-passive stretches* are stretches in which you assume a position and hold it for an extended period of time, using an external force such as your hands or strap or some type of stationary support such as a chair or a dancer's barre. Because this type of stretch is so accessible and straightforward, I choose to recommend it in this book.
- ✔ *Static-active stretches* are more advanced positions in which you stretch one muscle by contracting the opposing muscle (for example, stretching your hamstring by holding your extended leg as high off the ground as you can).

Although this stretching technique is highly effective when it comes to improving sports performance (see Chapter 12 for sports-specific stretches), it requires a more advanced level of strength and balance, which usually comes after a few months of routine stretching sessions.

Dynamic stretches

Simply put, dynamic stretching is a stretching technique that involves movement. When performing a dynamic stretch you simply use the weight of a portion of your body, such as a limb, to help overcome inertia in a tight muscle. You gently control the twisting of your torso or the swinging of your arms or legs in a movement that approaches the limit of your range of motion. The key word in that last sentence is *control* — dynamic stretches shouldn't be executed by bouncing or jerking. Think of your twisting or swinging motions as purposeful movements, almost like choreography.

A dynamic stretch that's being repeatedly forced beyond a comfortable range of motion is called a *ballistic* stretch. Ballistic stretching can be painful, counterproductive, and even cause injury. Bent over toe touching with a bouncing movement is a good example and is usually used by athletes who want to increase their range of motion. This type of stretching isn't used in this book.

 Dynamic stretches should also develop progressively. Start moving through the stretch slowly and with a small range of motion. Gradually increase the range of motion until, eventually, after 8 to 12 repetitions, the move has reached its full range of motion and maximum controlled pace.

When One Just Ain't Enough: Stretching with a Partner

A helpful, caring partner can be the ultimate stretching prop (for more info on props, see Chapter 3). A partner can

- ✓ Gently urge you deeper into a position than you may be able to do yourself
- ✓ Help you get far more out of your flexibility routine than you may be able to on your own

Nevertheless, there are some disadvantages:

- ✓ Your partner can't feel what you feel every moment.
- ✓ Your partner can't respond to your discomfort as quickly as you may like.
- ✓ Your partner may force you into a deeper position than you're ready for.
- ✓ Your partner can move you too quickly, which can initiate the stretch reflex (see "Static stretches" earlier in the chapter for more info on the stretch reflex).

 These instances can be a source of accidental injury, so maintain consistent communication with your partner to avoid uncomfortable situations.

In addition, using a partner is ideal for two types of stretches: isometric stretching and PNF stretching. Although I don't describe any of these types of exercises in this book, more advanced exercisers can adapt these techniques to the stretches I describe for beginners. Check out the next sections for the lowdown on these types of partner stretches.

Isometric stretching

Isometric stretching is a type of static stretch in which you tense a muscle in order to reduce tension in it. Sounds counterintuitive, doesn't it? Think of it as stretching in reverse.

The word *isometric* is comprised of the prefix "iso" (same) with "metric" (distance), indicating that in this type of exercise the length of the muscle doesn't change as a result of the flexing of a joint.

One of the best ways to perform an isometric stretch is to have a partner apply resistance against the muscle you want to stretch. For example, have a partner hold your extended leg up while you try to push it back down to the ground. Tensing your hamstring against that resistance actually reduces tension in the hamstring muscle. Plus, an extra added bonus of this type of stretching is that you can actually increase strength (a little) in the muscles you contract.

Static-isometric-static stretching

Proprioceptive neuromuscular facilitation (PNF) stretching is a big, fat phrase that means a static stretch, followed by an isometric stretch, followed by a deeper static stretch. In fact, PNF isn't really a type of stretch at all; it's more properly a stretching technique.

After comfortably holding a static stretch, your partner can add resistance to create an isometric stretch (see preceding section). The big payoff comes when the isometric stretch is released, and then after 10 to 15 seconds, your partner helps you move even deeper into the stretch than you were in the initial passive stretch. This addition is only made possible because of the concentrated stretch provided by the isometric stretch. But the end result is a more thorough stretch than you would ever have been able to achieve on your own.

I don't recommend PNF stretching (or isometric stretching for that matter) for children or anyone who may still be growing. Also, this type of stretch shouldn't be performed on a given muscle group more than once a day, or ideally, once per 36-hour period.

The Science of Stretching

This entire book is based on the miraculous capability of our bodies to adapt to the physical demands placed on them. Before you can use stretching to your benefit, you need to understand how it works, how it nurtures you, and how to maintain your body through stretching. No machine created has the awesome regenerative capability of the human body, so it's up to you to figure out how to properly take care of yourself and use stretching in that process.

What happens inside my muscles when I stretch them?

Visualizing and knowing what your body is doing while you're stretching is just as important as visualizing and knowing what muscle you're using when you're lifting weights (see Chapter 3 on testing your flexibility). So begins your science lesson for today . . . and, if you're anything like me, you have little interest in science, so I'll try to be brief and get right to the point!

The stretching of a muscle begins with the most elementary unit in the muscle fiber — the *sarcomere*. As the sarcomere is stretched, the overlap of the myofilaments decreases, allowing the muscle fiber to elongate (Whew! Now that's a mouthful). At that point, the surrounding connective tissue gives way to the force of your stretch and it also stretches. In other words, the greater number of myofilaments you can stretch, the greater flexibility you have in the muscle.

What is flexibility?

Flexibility is the extent to which your body is able to bend — without breaking or injury. So when you get right down to it, flexibility is a function of the number of muscle fibers you have been able to coerce into lengthening and the number of them you can *keep* lengthened.

Flexibility occurs when an electrical signal transmits from a nerve into the muscle fibers and stimulates the flow of calcium, causing the sarcomere to shorten, which generates force. When billions of sarcomeres in the muscle shorten all at once, the result is a total and complete contraction of the entire muscle fiber. Think of muscle fibers as being digital — they're either contracted or they're not. On/Off. But if there's no such thing as a partially contracted muscle fiber, how does the force of a muscle contraction vary in strength from strong to weak? Strength is a function of total muscle fibers involved — the greater the demand, the larger number of muscle fibers recruited to do the work.

Likewise, the length of the stretched muscle depends on the number of stretched fibers, which means that the more precise and thorough your stretching movements are — the more fibers you can involve — the greater benefit you receive from them.

How can I keep my muscles and joints stretched?

If you don't take your flexibility for granted, you can keep your muscle and joints stretched. Muscles are naturally inclined to contract for their own protection, so the only way to keep them elongated, and to keep your connective tissue lengthened, is to regularly stretch them. Remember, when it comes to stretching, the old saying "use it or lose it" truly applies.

Chapter 2

Preparing for a More Flexible You

. . . .

In This Chapter

▶ Identifying what you need to get started

▶ Personalizing your stretches with props

▶ Knowing how to stay injury free

▶ Getting the most out of your stretching program through proper form

▶ Taking a minute to relax

. . . .

The more you know about your body, the more power you have to improve your flexibility. I'm not saying you have to take a course in kinesiology or know where all 650 muscles in your body attach (whew!), but a quick refresher course in the major muscle groups of your body may help you identify if the stretch is coming from the right place and also help you understand *why* you feel the stretch as you move through the exercises.

Even though you're getting this lesson as the first step in flexibility training, before you start stretching you should look at the anatomy drawings in Chapters 4–7. They provide a visual reference of the *origin* (where the muscle starts) and the *insertion* (where the muscle attaches) of the major muscles. These pictures help you understand why placing your body in a certain position stretches certain muscles and how to stretch those muscles most effectively.

After you have a general knowledge of the muscles in your body, you're one step closer to a more flexible you!

Getting Your Stretch On: The How To's of Stretching

Even if you consider stretching simple and easy, you have to give yourself every advantage to make your stretching experience successful. The following sections give you a wealth of knowledge and tips to ensure that your flexibility program is totally tight . . . I mean, you know, very effective.

Creating space fit for stretching

One of the most fundamental and most often overlooked aspects of flexibility training (as with most workout programs) is commitment, and true commitment is reflected both externally — by creating a specific, special place to stretch — and internally — getting yourself into the right frame of mind.

If you've ever been to a yoga class, you know what I mean by getting in the right frame of mind (an open neat space with soft, serene music and a teacher who whispers). All these external and internal factors add up to a better stretching experience, so you can look forward to your next stretching session even more.

Organizing your surroundings

Here are a few things you can do to keep your space (external factor) uncluttered:

- **Establish a space large enough to extend your body fully.** You may have to move some of the furniture around you, but there's nothing more annoying than having to move things while you're stretching. Get it taken care of ahead of time and you won't have to deal with the interruption while you're stretching.

- **Make the room warm.** An ideal stretching room is a warm room because your muscles respond more to stretching when they're warm. So don't crank up the air conditioner just because you hate to sweat.

Because stretching can't be hurried or rushed, you have to move slowly and deliberately. Such an attitude should also be reflected in your mental approach (next section).

Collecting your thoughts

Here are a few things you can do to keep your mind (internal factor) uncluttered:

- **Relaxing music:** You can buy instrumental or relaxation CDs that definitely allow you to unwind more easily and help you have a great mind/body experience.

- **Planning ahead:** Make sure that your workout isn't interrupted. Turn off the phone, put your Blackberry where you can't see it, and tell your kids you've moved away to join the circus. (Okay, maybe not the last one. Just say interruptions are for emergencies only!)

Getting dressed

Unlike in packed, sweaty group exercise classes, the optimum outfit for stretching isn't one that makes you look good, it's one that makes you *feel* good. And what I find makes me feel good is clothes that don't get in the way. Always wear comfortable clothing that doesn't bind or restrict your movement but that still enables you to see your body so you can tell what you're actually doing.

Ballet dancers wear leotards and tights so they can see if their back is arched or straight and the same principle applies for stretching . . . you have to be able to see what your body is doing so you can focus on specific muscles. Therefore, I find a tank top and a pair of tights or a nice fitting T-shirt with shorts works best when I'm stretching.

Give Yourself Props! How to Personalize Each Stretch

A prop isn't just part of a movie set anymore. A prop can be used for stretching and is something such as a strap, a towel, a chair, or a block that you can use to make a stretch more comfortable, accessible, and even more effective (see Chapter 17 for more prop ideas). Props have a wide variety of benefits:

- Beginners and the less flexible can use them to perform a stretch that they may otherwise not be able to manage.

- By providing support and reducing tension, props can help you position your body more correctly, which not only helps make your stretches as deep and effective as possible but also helps decrease the chance of injury.

- For more experienced exercisers, props allow you to deepen and intensify the stretch.

I recommend using props for any stretch that you want to help make more comfortable, well balanced, and tension free. The next sections include some of my favorite props that enhance your stretching experience. You can also find more props in Chapter 17. The props in that chapter are handy things that you should have lying around the house!

Strap or towel

A *stretching strap* is a length of slightly elastic material that you can use to increase your reach. Many brands have several loops in which you can place your hands or feet to customize the strap to your height and flexibility. This elasticity helps increase your chance of achieving a comfortable, passive static stretch for a variety of muscles. No matter what the stretch, a strap can also help keep your upper back relaxed, which keeps your spine in neutral position and avoids scrunching or rounding of your back.

A *yoga strap* is another prop that you can use and it's usually made of cotton and comes in 6- or 8-foot lengths. Yoga straps typically don't have the loops usually found on stretching straps. Instead, a yoga strap has a buckle that allows you to create a loop in one end of the strap. The 6-foot strap will probably be long enough for most of you, but if you're over 6 feet tall, you may want to try the 8-foot length. These straps are easy to find on the Internet or at a local yoga center.

A towel isn't as customizable as a stretching strap or a yoga strap, but it's a great substitute if neither of the straps is available or if you simply don't want to spend the money. A hand towel is a little small, so use a gym towel or small bath towel to have plenty of length to work with. But if you plan on making stretching a permanent part of your fitness routine (which I highly recommend), purchase a strap of your own. It's a small investment of less than ten bucks, and you won't regret it.

Blocks

Using a yoga block under your buttocks, feet, or hands helps you maintain proper body alignment during stretches so you can focus on deepening your stretch without pain. The cost of one block is usually around $10, and you can find blocks at most yoga studios or your local superstore.

If you love to shop online, hop on the Internet and type in *yoga props* and choose from the nearly one million sites that pop up.

Also, if you don't want to invest in a block just yet, I bet you have a phone book sitting around the house. Even sitting on a folded towel helps give you the lift off the floor.

Chair

A chair can add stability to standing stretches and can also help you get into stretches that require stress-free support of your torso. A chair is particularly useful for seniors or anyone with mobility issues. It's also one of the best props to help a sedentary person get started with a flexibility program. For stretches that use a chair, check out Chapter 8 for total body workouts, Chapter 10 for stretches during the workday, and Chapter 15 — stretches for seniors.

Make sure to use a sturdy chair without arms or wheels and that's not too cushy.

Swiss ball

No, the Swiss ball isn't a ball of cheese. It's similar to the chair, but it allows you to get into some stretches more comfortably than if you had to lie down on the floor. Lying with your tummy on the ball is great for stretching out your lower back, and using the Swiss ball to replace your chair at work helps you strengthen your core as you stretch out your legs and back. For another example of a ball stretch, check out the chest stretch in Chapter 14.

If you've never used a stretching ball before or if you just want some stretches that use the Swiss ball, check out another book I wrote: *Exercise Balls For Dummies* (Wiley).

Foam roller

The *foam roller* is a lightweight cylinder that comes in many different sizes. When stretching, you can use the foam roller as a prop to make positions more comfortable by supporting your back or other body parts, thereby allowing you to keep good form and proper alignment.

Physical therapists and private trainers use this prop to improve balance, body awareness, and flexibility in their patients. But what really makes the foam roller unique from other props is that you can actually use it to release muscular tension and pain.

Imagine a rubber band that has a knot in it — no matter how much you stretch that rubber band you'll never get rid of the knot. Everyone gets a muscle with a knot (localized tightness often caused by tension or overuse) and sometimes stretching isn't enough. That's where the foam roller comes in handy.

By positioning your body to slowly roll on the foam roller you can actually release the knots in your muscles. Here's a great example of how you use a foam roller to release tension in your back:

1. **Lie on the floor with your knees bent at a 90-degree angle and your feet flat on the floor.**

2. **Flatten your back by pressing your back into the floor and gently contracting your abdominal muscles and buttocks without raising your ribcage.**

3. **Repeat the same flat back position with a foam roller.**

   • Lie on the roller with hips and knees flexed and feet flat on the floor.

   • Keep your back flat and in contact with the roam roller.

4. **Add a few movements to your stable core position by slowly rolling your body back and forth while the foam roller is pressing into your back.**

5. **To strengthen your core, raise one leg while maintaining a neutral spine and lower the leg and raise the other leg.**

   Alternate raising and lowering your legs, making sure to keep your back in contact with the foam roller at all times.

The cost of a foam roller is about $25 — a heck of a lot cheaper than a massage or a visit to your chiropractor!

Refraining from Hurting Yourself

Some of the key points to stretching are to stay relaxed and comfortable and to enjoy yourself. But you also need to follow a few simple guidelines before you stretch. These strategies and techniques ensure that you take care of your body, prevent injuries, and get the most out of your flexibility training.

Warm-up

The number-one rule with stretching is to warm up *before* you stretch! Many people think that stretching and warming up are synonymous, but stretching involves lengthening your muscles, while warming up means that you're elevating your core body temperature.

A muscle can't stretch properly if it's cold. Elevating your body temperature makes the process of extending and lengthening your muscles and the connective tissue around your muscles easier. These lengthenings and extensions reduce the chances of injury caused by stretching and actually increase the effectiveness of the stretch.

Here are some simple five-minute exercises to get those muscles warmed up:

- Performing jumping jacks
- Jumping rope
- Jogging in place
- Swimming laps
- Dancing around to your favorite song

I know this section probably shattered your conception of warming up, but now that you know the truth (that stretching and warming up describe two completely different processes), remember this: You can warm up without stretching, but you should never stretch without warming up.

For more information on how to integrate stretches into your warm-up, check out Chapter 11.

Go slowly

If stretching had a theme song it would be "The 59th Street Bridge Song (Feelin' Groovy)" by Simon and Garfunkel. You may know the words:

Slow down, you move too fast

You got to make the morning last

Just kicking down the cobblestones

Looking for fun and feelin' groovy

When you stretch you should move slowly; breathe and hold the stretch for at least 30 seconds. At first you may actually need to watch a clock to know how long 30 seconds is, but as you get more comfortable with stretching and more in tune with your body, you instinctively know how long to hold the stretch. For me, it's about four or five deep breaths. Keep your mind focused on the stretch and on breathing slowly and deeply. Don't think about all the things you have to do today or what you're going to cook for dinner, just stay focused on going slow and feelin' groovy!

To help prevent injuries, start each stretch in what I call the *comfort zone* — the point in the stretch where you just begin to feel mild tension in the muscle. Start out by stretching for 30 seconds or four to five slow, deep breaths before trying a second repetition. As you increase repetitions, it helps if you imagine every exhale you take as allowing you to move an inch deeper into the stretch. Believe it or not, the slower you go in the beginning, the more quickly you'll see results! See "Progress through the stretch" later in this chapter for more info on the progression.

Don't bounce

The second crucial guideline to keep in mind is *no bouncing!* Bouncing during your stretching actually causes damage to the muscle. Stretching a muscle quickly or forcefully makes your body kick into a natural protective mechanism called the stretch reflex — a nerve response to stress that tells the muscle to contract to protect itself. In other words, bouncing to help your muscles relax and let go can actually cause them to contract and get tighter.

And what's more, every time you forcefully bounce while in a stretch you actually create microscopic tears in the muscle fibers. You may feel like bouncing increases your flexibility immediately, but that's only because you have damaged the muscle. In the end, your body heals those little tears with scar tissue, which actually decreases your long-term flexibility, because scar tissue is far less flexible than muscle.

Progress through the stretch

I like to think of each stretch progressing through three different stages:

1. **Comfort zone:** The first 10 to 15 seconds

   This term describes the initial period of the stretch where you find a comfortable position, give yourself a body check, and make sure your alignment is good. You should also feel a mild tension in the muscle group that you're stretching.

2. **Relaxation zone:** The next 5 to 15 seconds

   This period in the stretch focuses on your breathing and relaxation — letting stress and tension melt away from both your body and mind. You may feel the stretch deepen slightly.

3. **Deep stretch zone:** The last 5 to 10 seconds

   You've now held the stretch for 20 to 30 seconds. Your body is relaxed, and you know that you're in correct position because you feel a slight tension precisely in the intended area. Remember you want to feel slight discomfort, not pain!

All the stretches in this book should be approached in the progressive fashion above. Never try to begin a stretch fully extended. Take your time and slowly and gradually move deeper with each breath, allowing the muscle to relax and giving your body the time to produce the correct neuromuscular response.

Remember to breathe

You may think that I am silly for telling you to breathe, but trust me; during a stretch (especially a hard one) you focus so hard that you forget to breathe and you tend to hold your breath instead. The only way to stretch a muscle fully is to relax and practice slow, rhythmic breathing. To simplify things, try to remember to exhale so your body automatically inhales. Don't make it any more complicated than that for right now. See "The Art of Breathing Correctly" later in this chapter for more information.

Know your limits

Stretching can help you understand both your possibilities and your limits. Stretching is supposed to be energizing and relaxing, not painful. Never do anything that hurts! You may not believe it right now, but flexibility training should *not* be painful. In fact, if you feel pain of any kind, let up on the stretch immediately.

Not everyone is able to do the perfect splits, and you don't need to. Stretching isn't a competition; it's about determining your current level of flexibility, whatever that may be, and improving on that foundation. Different people begin with different foundations. What matters most is that you're able to make yourself more flexible than you were. This increased flexibility can help improve your performance in your favorite sports and activities, and, by making movement more fluid, easy, and graceful, help enhance the overall quality of your life.

Maintaining Proper Body Alignment

Proper body alignment is your guarantee that you're getting the most out of your stretches. Why? Because when you maintain proper body alignment — back straight, shoulders down, chest lifted, abs tight — you optimize the mechanics of your body so your stretches are properly anchored and the muscle you're focusing on is fully lengthened. You also won't unintentionally put stress and strain on other parts of your body, which can be counterproductive to what you're trying to achieve. Pay attention to what every part of your body is doing.

Several studies suggest that a relationship exists between flexibility and posture. Researchers have found that imbalances in muscular development or tension can contribute to poor posture. For example, tight hamstrings can cause the pelvis to tilt up unnaturally, which can reduce the lumbar curve, exaggerate the thoracic curve, and possibly cause low back pain. This section explains how stretching can have a positive effect on posture and how proper posture can have a positive effect on stretching.

You may notice that one side of your body is more flexible than the other. This imbalance is very common, so don't worry about it — and be sure to not go easy on the side that is less flexible. Really focus and try to increase your range of motion until both sides are even.

Don't slouch (Darn it — Mom's right again)

Poor posture, or slouching, is unattractive, and it can lead to poor breathing, upper back tension, and inefficient movement. One common cause of slouching is shortened chest muscles and weak upper back muscles. The imbalance of the two pulls the shoulders forward.

The solution: stretching your chest and strengthening your back, which you find out how to do in Chapters 4 and 8. And in the meantime, try to be aware of your posture and make sure that you stand erect and sit up straight.

Introducing the neutral spine

Throughout this book I remind you to find or maintain *neutral spine*. You may be wondering what the heck that means but just remember you have a natural curve in your back when you relax. So I'm making sure that you don't exaggerate or minimize the way your spine is naturally shaped.

Your spine has four natural curves:

1. The cervical (the curve in your neck)
2. The thoracic (the slightly rounded shape in your upper back)
3. The lumbar (the sway of your lower back)
4. The sacrum (the tilt of your pelvic region)

In flexibility training, neutral spine has three positions: lying on your back, sitting, and standing. Start each stretch in neutral spine because incorrect spinal position not only diminishes the effectiveness of the stretch but also promotes muscular imbalance and bad posture. Every time you start in correct alignment you retrain your muscles to properly support your spine.

Although exercising is excellent therapy for your spine, many people make simple but crucial mistakes in the position of their spine while exercising. These mistakes can place a great deal of stress on the spine. Some of the most common are

- Decreasing the curve in the lower back by "tucking" the pelvis under
- Excessively arching the back by tilting the pelvis backward
- Exaggerating the thoracic curve by rounding the shoulders forward and tightening the shoulder muscles
- Lifting and opening the rib cage while reaching overhead
- Forgetting that the neck is actually part of your spine
- Letting the chin drop down or the head jut forward

Positioning your pelvis

The area of the pelvis is the main hinge between the torso and the lower body, so correct positioning of the pelvis is crucial for lower body stretches involving the hips, thighs, and buttocks. Because these large muscles are all attached in one way or another to the pelvis, incorrect positioning of the pelvis can cause these lower body stretches to be inefficient or even actually counterproductive.

To find the proper pelvic position that you should maintain while you're stretching, try standing in front of a mirror and turning sideways. Stand up tall so your body is in a straight line from head to toe. This position is the correct position you want to have in your pelvis.

You *don't* want to do the following:

✔ Tilt your pelvis forward — described as "tucking your pelvis under"

✔ Arch your back and let your buttocks stick out

The Art of Breathing Correctly

Believe it or not, you breathe in and out more than 20,000 times a day, and yet, most of the time you do it incorrectly. I can hear you asking, "How is it possible to breathe wrong? Air goes in; air goes out. How can something so simple be any more complicated?" Well, due to poor posture or lack of body awareness, you end up using the wrong muscles to breathe. The end result is shallow, ineffective breathing that robs you of all the full benefits of your breath. Poor posture — with a rounded back, dropped shoulders, and a forward head — reduces the ability of the diaphragm to contract and the ribs to expand to their full potential.

The lung itself has no muscles, so it's totally dependent on the muscles around it to create the respiratory process of inhaling and exhaling. This can happen two ways: by using the muscles that lift and lower the ribcage or by using the muscles of the diaphragm.

Unfortunately, most people use the shoulder and chest muscles to facilitate the respiratory process of inhaling and exhaling. Although these muscles are large and powerful, breathing isn't really what they were designed for. Instead, the primary location of the movement of respiration should be the diaphragm, which only has one function: breathing.

Here are some healthy breathing tips that you can find an example of in Chapter 8:

✔ Inhale through your nose, filling your chest with air and letting your belly expand. This technique allows your nose to filter and warm the air before your body uses it.

✔ Make sure that your shoulders stay relaxed and don't raise up around your ears when you're breathing.

✔ Exhale through your mouth, consciously using your deep abdominal muscles and diaphragm to push the air out (belly will deflate).

Just remember, to get all these wonderful benefits, you need to breathe the way your body was designed — from your core.

Relaxing and Letting Go

One of the most important benefits of stretching is its ability to promote relaxation not only of your body but also of your mind and spirit. The slow, methodical movements in a good flexibility program provide gentle movements as you position your body for the next stretch, followed by periods of quiet stillness as you hold the stretch. Concentrated focus on the muscles you're stretching helps block out other stress-inducing thoughts (you know, those thoughts of your schedule, your finances, your kids, and so on). In this way, stretching can not only lengthen your muscles but also expand your mental horizon.

When you stretch, keep the following in mind:

- You should feel slight tension in the muscle that you intend to stretch. This tension should definitely not cross the line into pain or discomfort.

- You should feel a stretch only in the intended muscle, never in a joint. Pain in your joints signals irritation in the joint, so you definitely want to let up if that happens.

- Your body should be in a position that's relaxed and totally tension free. If your body feels awkward or tense, modify the stretch, or use a prop such as a strap or block (covered earlier in this chapter) so you can focus on the intended muscle.

- Stretching should be a positive experience, not a form of self-torture.

Throughout this book I give you several different stretches for each muscle group. If one doesn't seem to fit your body, try one that feels more comfortable.

Chapter 3

Testing Your Flexibility to Establish Your Stretching Routine

In This Chapter

▶ Understanding what factors affect your flexibility

▶ Determining your own flexibility through self-testing

▶ Recording your results and tracking your improvements

Some people are fast runners; some people are good singers; some people are flexible — and some people aren't. But when it comes to flexibility, it's really a question of degrees. While it's important to have a healthy range of motion in all your muscles and joints just to live a balanced, healthy, injury-free life, being superflexible is really only necessary if you're a professional dancer or gymnast (so don't get discouraged if you can't put your foot behind your head!). This chapter is designed to help you determine how flexible you really are and which areas of your body need the most attention so you can become as flexible as can be.

Coming to Terms with the Factors of Flexibility

Before you can set a reasonable goal, you need to understand what's achievable and what isn't. Everyone can't get a job with the Cirque du Soleil or do the splits, but not everyone should for the simple reason that not every *body* is designed to bend that way.

Several factors determine your flexibility, and you can change some of those factors and some you can't. But before you can work on making improvements in your flexible status, you have to be realistic. In the following sections, I present several areas of the body that you can improve on. Take a look at the factors in each category to see what differences you can make in your body with flexibility. And then check out the things that you can't change.

What you can change

Flexibility is the ability of your body to move through the required range of motion to perform the activity at hand. But what happens if you don't have flexibility in your body? You may be uncoordinated or tense, but here are some factors you can positively alter in your life to get the most out of your flexibility training:

✔ **Muscle tension:** If a muscle is tense or in a state of contraction then it can't increase in flexibility. It's important to be in a state of relaxation to get the full benefits of stretching (see Chapter 2 for tips on relaxing).

✔ **Lack of coordination and body awareness:** Lack of coordination can limit your ability to stretch the targeted muscle, therefore diminishing the effectiveness of the stretch. You have to pay attention to what's happening to your muscles as you stretch and you have to be mindful of your movement, all the while continually improving your form.

✔ **Lifestyle:** Eat right, exercise regularly, and adhere to your flexibility training. Practice makes perfect, and that advice applies to becoming more flexible, too.

✔ **Warming up:** You need to make sure to warm up your muscles *before* you stretch. When a muscle and the connective tissue around that muscle are warm they stretch more easily and with less resistance — and you get more benefit from your stretching routines. Check out Chapter 11 for some ways to warm up properly.

✔ **Your attitude:** You'll never see your best results without a positive attitude. Of course that philosophy applies to more in life than just stretching, but focus on flexibility training for now.

What you can't change

To avoid any unrealistic expectations, remember that there are some physical factors that everyone has in common that simply can't be changed. Yes, genetics do play a big part in individual flexibility, so I guess it's okay to blame your family for this one . . . sorry mom!

✔ **Your gender:** Research indicates that, in general, women are more flexible than men. One reason could be because of bone structure because, for example, women usually have broader and shallower hips, which give them a potential for greater range of motion in the pelvic area.

✔ **Your age:** The aging process diminishes normal muscle function, including strength, endurance, and flexibility. Lost muscle mass is replaced with fat and collagen. Collagen is the main component in connective tissue and is highly inflexible. Although aging is, of course, inevitable, you can greatly slow down this process with your lifestyle choices, such as eating right, exercising, and stretching regularly!

✔ **Elasticity of connective tissue in muscles or joints:** Don't think of flexibility in terms of your whole body; think in terms of the range of motion of each joint. And each of the joints in your body is made up of bones, muscles, and three types of connective tissue:

  • **Tendons:** Tendons connect muscle to bone, and they drag the bone along when the muscle moves. Firm, strong tendons are a good thing because without them your muscles would be inefficient and unstable. You don't focus on stretching the tendons in this book.

  • **Ligaments:** Ligaments connect bone to bone (such as the bones in your knees and in your elbows) and play a large role in the stability of a joint and how much range of motion is possible in that joint. Because you don't want wiggly knees or elbows, you don't want to stretch your ligaments, either.

  • **Fascia:** This tissue is the rest of the connective tissue in your body. You can find fascia under the skin, deep in your body surrounding your organs and within your muscles, holding the fibers of the muscle together in a compact, efficient bunch.

    As much as 30 percent of a muscle is fascia, but the precise percentage is determined solely by genetics, so the amount of fascia in your muscles can play a large role in how tight or flexible your muscles can be. If you were born with a high percentage of fascia in your muscles, chances are you will be less flexible overall.

✔ **Your bone and joint structure limitations:** You can thank Mom and Dad for your bone structure. Plain and simple, some people's joints allow more range of motion than others. Get over it. Just like your childhood.

Testing Yourself Before (and While, and After) You Go Gumby-Like

The very best motivation to stick with an exercise program is seeing results, which is why I've developed the flexibility self-test I include in the next section. The test helps you accomplish two important goals:

✔ **Indicates where you're tight and where your imbalances may be so you know where to focus your stretching program:** For example, by doing this self-test, you may discover that your quadriceps (muscles in the front of your thigh) are tight but you have a healthy range of motion in your hamstrings (muscles in the back of your thigh). Eventually this imbalance between these two opposing muscle groups may lead to an injury. Thanks to this self-test you now have the information to prevent that from happening by putting more time and effort into stretching your quadriceps and less on your hamstrings.

Another common imbalance that leads to injury or postural problems is being tighter on one side of your body than the other. That's why in this self-test you document your range of motion on both the right and left sides of your body. If you were to discover that your left shoulder has more range of motion than your right shoulder, you can put a little more time into stretching your right shoulder.

✔ **Records and tracks your increases in flexibility over time:** The only way to tell how far you've come is to know precisely where you started. And the only way to know how far you've gotten is to measure your progress regularly. Performing this self-test before you begin your flexibility training gives you a good idea of your initial flexibility level.

Measure yourself every six weeks to see how well you're doing. And nothing breeds success like success. The more you find yourself improving, the more motivated you will be to keep up the good work!

Developing increased flexibility doesn't happen overnight. You need to set realistic goals, and start with easy exercises before moving on to more advanced ones. Testing is for recording progress, not for competing. No two people are alike. Some people may see results more quickly and dramatically than others, but as long as you're seeing improvement and enjoying yourself, you have a much better chance of making stretching a lifelong program.

The self-test takes about 20 minutes to complete, so make sure to have enough time to complete the test. As you test yourself more often and get more familiar with the stretches, the time will decrease. To get started, you need the following:

✔ Comfortable, loose fitting clothes

✔ Mat or carpeted floor — you need a space large enough to lie down comfortably

✔ Firm chair or exercise bench

✔ Stretching table or your bed

✔ Flexibility Evaluation Worksheet (included at the end of this chapter)

✔ Pen or pencil

✔ A towel or stretching strap — for a more detailed description of what type of strap, check out Chapter 2

If you're really dedicated to increasing your flexibility and you have made a commitment to stick with your stretching program, I suggest investing a few dollars and purchasing your own stretching strap — it will be well worth the money. Until then, just use a small bath towel or gym towel.

Putting Your Legs Where Your Head Is . . . Not: The Flexibility Self-Test

Performing a stretch that involves more than one muscle group makes it difficult to determine which muscle is tight or which ones cause limited range of motion. For example, you may have heard of the "sit and reach" test — where you sit on the floor with your legs straight out in front of you, and you bend forward while someone measures with a ruler how far you can reach toward your toes (you may have done this test in high school; it's a popular test on Fitness Day). Even though this test is common for flexibility, I'm not a big fan of it because it gives you very little information — it tells you if your muscles are tight or not, but it doesn't tell you which muscles; is it your lower back, your hamstrings, or your calves that are tight? Who knows?

So my test is different. My stretch test isolates individual muscles to give you the most useful information possible to design your own customized stretching program. At first, the following sections of stretches may seem like a lot, but unfortunately there's no such thing as just a few moves to determine flexibility.

After you completed the self-test, you know exactly what muscles in your body need the most attention. At that point, you can head to the chapter in this book that contains specific stretches for the areas you want to work and then choose the exercise(s) that feels most comfortable for your body.

Also, you may notice that most of the stretches test both the right and left sides of your body. It's not uncommon to have one side more flexible than the other, which creates an imbalance, but it's important to try to get both sides of your body equal in flexibility for symmetry, balance, and injury prevention, and this test helps you achieve that goal.

Before you start, I want to give you a few pointers:

- You get better results if you warm up before you attempt these tests. You can head to Chapter 11 for some simple warm-up exercises. I recommend doing the same warm-up routine every time you do this stretch test — that way you get more consistent and accurate results.

- When you retest to check your progress, make sure that you always test in similar situations: time of day, amount of warm-up, workout schedule, and so on.

- In the section "Flexibility Self-Evaluation Worksheet," I include a worksheet for recording your performance on each of the stretches in this chapter. Each stretch isolates a specific area.

As you perform the stretch, imagine a large clock around you with the center of the clock pinned to the axis of the stretch. For instance, when standing up and twisting, the clock would be on the ground, directly beneath the centerline of your body — the axis around which you are stretching. Midnight would be looking straight ahead. If you're sitting on the ground leaning forward, the clock would be centered on your hip, the axis of your stretch. Midnight would be when you're sitting up straight.

✔ Because this is only an assessment, not an attempt to increase your range of motion, don't hold the stretches for an extended period of time. Just get into the correct position, inhale deeply and as you exhale make a note of your position as it corresponds to the hands on a clock, and write in down on your worksheet.

Let the testing begin!

Neck

The chin-to-chest neck stretch gives you an idea of how tight the muscles are in your neck. To test the muscles in this area, stretch following the steps below:

1. **Sit up tall in a chair with your back straight, arms at your sides, and your shoulders down.**

   Don't round your back forward.

2. **Inhale and as you exhale drop your chin down toward your chest, as shown in Figure 3-1.**

3. **Make a note on your Flexibility Self-Evaluation Worksheet at what place on the clock face the top of your head points.**

   Imagine that the clock face is centered on the outside of your shoulder.

   - 1:00 is tight.

   - 2:00 is a healthy range of motion.

   - 3:00 is very flexible.

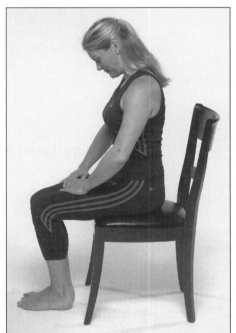

Figure 3-1:
Testing the flexibility of the back of your neck.

Shoulders

This simple movement can tell you a lot about the range of motion in your shoulders. To do this test stretch, follow these steps:

1. **Stand up tall with your back straight, your abdominals lifted, your shoulders down, and your arms to your side.**

2. **Inhale and as you exhale lift your right arm straight forward, moving it as far overhead as you can (Figure 3-2).**

   Remember to keep your shoulders down and don't let your back arch. Stop moving if you feel pain in your shoulder.

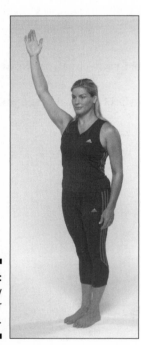

Figure 3-2:
A flexibility test for your shoulders.

3. **Make a note on your Flexibility Self-Evaluation Worksheet at what place on the clock face your hand points.**

   - 10:00 is tight.

   - 12:00 is a healthy range of motion.

   - 1:00 is very flexible.

4. **Repeat this stretch with your left arm and mark your results on the worksheet.**

   - 2:00 is tight.

   - 12:00 is a healthy range of motion.

   - 11:00 is very flexible.

Chest

To test the flexibility of your chest, follow these steps:

1. **Stand up tall with your back straight, your abdominals lifted, your shoulders down, and your arms at your sides.**

2. **Inhale and bring your arms straight out in front of you at chest height.**

3. **Exhale and open your arms to the side (palms facing forward) as far as you can without arching your back (see Figure 3-3).**

   Keep your shoulder blades down and stable.

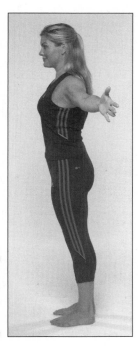

Figure 3-3: The flexibility test for your chest.

4. **Make a note on your worksheet at what place on the clock your hands point.**
   - 10:00 and 2:00 are tight.
   - 9:00 and 3:00 are a healthy range of motion.
   - 8:00 and 4:00 are very flexible.

Trunk

A healthy back has a balanced range of motion in four directions: forward, side, rotation, and back. Isolating the muscles of your trunk can be difficult because many muscles are involved in the complex movement of your spine; therefore, there are four test stretches in this section to measure the range of motion in your trunk as a whole.

Seated rotation

To do this test stretch, follow these steps:

1. **Sit up tall in a chair with your back straight, your abdominals lifted, and your shoulders down.**

2. **Place your left arm on the outside of your right thigh and your right hand on the back seat of your chair.**

   This position helps you turn your upper body at the waist in the next step.

3. **Inhale and as you exhale twist at your waist as if you were trying to look behind you.**

   This position is shown in Figure 3-4. Remember to keep both shoulders down and to look out in front of you, not at the floor.

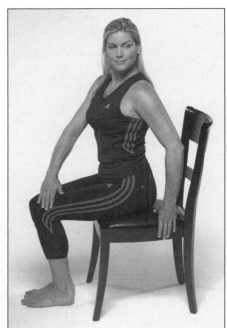

Figure 3-4:
Testing your
flexibility
with the
seated
rotation.

4. **Make a note on the Flexibility Self-Evaluation Worksheet at what place on the clock your chest faces.**

   - 1:00 is tight.

   - 2:00 is a healthy range of motion.

   - 3:00 is very flexible.

5. **Repeat this stretch by rotating to your left side and record the results on your worksheet.**

   - 11:00 is tight.

   - 10:00 is a healthy range of motion.

   - 9:00 is very flexible.

Standing side bend

To do this test stretch, follow these steps:

1. **Stand with your feet hip-width apart and your back straight, abdominals lifted, and your shoulders down.**

2. **Place your right hand overhead and your left arm to your side (see Figure 3-5a).**

3. **Inhale and as you exhale bend to the left side, reaching the fingers on your left hand down the side of your leg (Figure 3-5b).**

   Try to keep your shoulders and hips facing the front, avoiding even the slightest rotation in the spine.

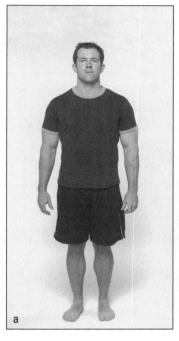 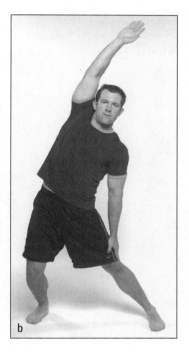

Figure 3-5: Flexibility test for lateral trunk movement.

a

b

4. **Make a note on the Flexibility Self-Evaluation Worksheet at what place on the clock face the top of your head points to.**

   • 1:00 is tight

   • 2:00 is healthy range of motion

   • 3:00 is very flexible

5. **Repeat this stretch on your other side (to stretch the left side).**

   • 11:00 is tight

   • 10:00 is healthy range of motion

   • 9:00 is very flexible

Seated forward bend

A tight upper or lower back limits your range of motion. To do this test stretch, follow these steps:

1. **Sit on a chair with your feet flat on the floor (see Figure 3-6a).**

2. **Inhale and as you exhale round forward a far as you comfortably can, bending at your hips (Figure 3-6b).**

3. **Make a note on the Flexibility Self-Evaluation Worksheet at what place on the clock face the back of your head points to.**

   - 1:00 is tight.

   - 2:00 is healthy range of motion.

   - 3:00 is very flexible.

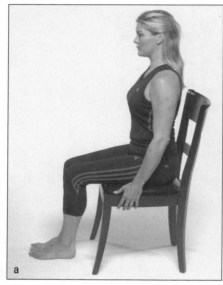
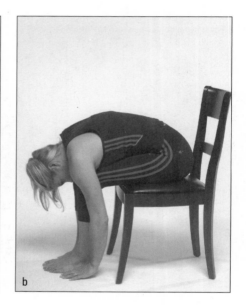

Figure 3-6: Flexibility test for trunk forward flexion.

Standing back extension

You may have tight abdominals if this stretch is difficult. To do this test stretch, follow these steps:

1. **Stand up tall with your back straight, your abdominals lifted, and your shoulders down with your arms to your sides and your feet apart.**

2. **Inhale and as you exhale move your shoulders back, lifting your chest and eyes toward the ceiling without compressing your lower back.**

   Think of keeping your spine long. Figure 3-7 shows you how to keep from compressing your back. You can also put your hands on your lower back for support.

3. **Make a note on your worksheet at what point on the clock your head stops moving.**

   Between 12:00 and 11:00 is tight.

   Between 11:00 and 10:00 is a healthy range of motion.

   Between 10:00 and 9:00 is very flexible.

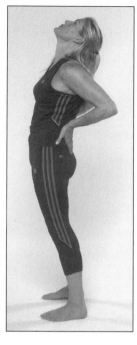

Figure 3-7:
Using the back extension to test your trunk's flexibility.

Quadriceps

This stretch tests the flexibility in your quadriceps (front of your thighs). Knowing where your tightness lies allows you to focus on stretches that improve your range of motion in this muscle group.

To stretch your quads, follow these steps:

1. **Stand up tall and place your left hand on a stable surface.**

   Your surface can be a chair, wall, doorway, or fence — anything that's sturdy and helps you keep your balance in the next steps.

2. **Inhale and lift your right foot behind you and grab hold of your ankle or the top of your foot with your right hand (see Figure 3-8).**

3. **Exhale and gently move your knee back, trying to line it up next to your left knee.**

   Don't force your heel to touch your right buttocks.

4. **Make a note on your Flexibility Self-Evaluation Worksheet at what place on the clock your knee points.**

   8:00 is very tight.

   7:00 is tight.

   6:00 is good flexibility.

5. **Repeat this stretch on your left side.**

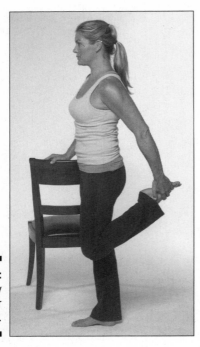

Figure 3-8:
A flexibility test for your quads.

Hamstrings

To do this test stretch, you need a towel or stretching strap. For more information about what type of strap to use check out Chapter 2 and read the discussion on props. Then follow these steps:

1. **Lie down on the floor with your legs straight out in front of you and your arms to your sides.**

2. **Bring your right foot toward your chest and wrap a strap or towel around the arch of your foot (see Figure 3-9).**

3. **Inhale and as you exhale extend your right leg toward the ceiling, as shown in Figure 3-9.**

   Try to keep your right leg as straight as possible and your hips on the floor. If it's more comfortable for you, you can bend your left leg so that your foot is on the floor but it's important to try to keep your right leg straight, even if it is not straight up to the ceiling. Remember, you are only evaluating your flexibility, so it's okay if your leg does not go very high. Keep working at it and stretch regularly and you'll soon see improvement.

4. **Make a note on your worksheet at what point your foot stops.**

   10:00 is tight.

   12:00 is a healthy range of motion.

   1:00 is very flexible.

5. **Repeat this stretch with your left leg and record those results on your worksheet, too.**

Groin

Groin pulls are often related to improper stretching or tight adductors, and this test reflects your flexibility in your *adductors* (inner thigh muscles).

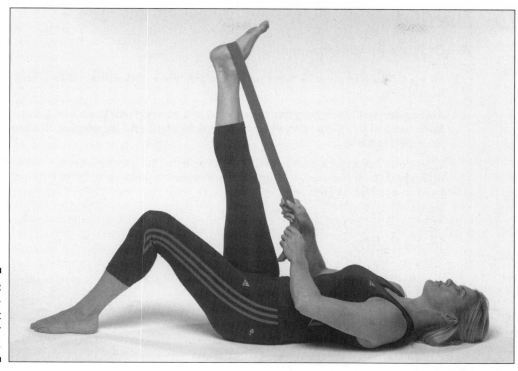

Figure 3-9:
The flexibility test for your hamstrings.

This area is often tighter in men than in women because women usually have broader and shallower hips, which give them a potential for greater range of motion in this area.

To do this test stretch, follow these steps:

1. **Lie down on the floor with your legs straight out in front of you and your arms to your sides.**

2. **Inhale and as you exhale move your legs out to the side as far as you comfortably can.**

   Remember when you were little and you used to make snow angels? You move your legs out like you were making an angel but without moving your arms. See Figure 3-10 for additional help.

3. **Make a note on your worksheet at what place on the clock your feet point.**

   7:00 and 5:00 are tight.

   8:00 and 4:00 are healthy range of motion.

   9:00 and 3:00 are very flexible.

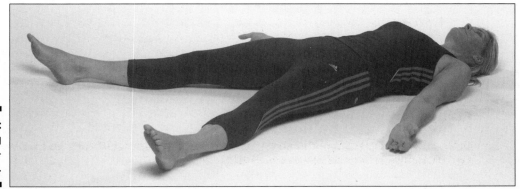

Figure 3-10:
The lying groin flexibility test.

Buttocks

To do this test stretch, follow these steps:

1. **Sit up tall in a chair with your back straight, your abdominals lifted, and your shoulders down.**

2. **Place your left ankle on your right quad just above your knee and gently press your knee toward the floor with your left hand as you bend forward at the hip and tilt your pelvis back.**

   Check out Figure 3-11 if you need help visualizing this stretch. Remember to keep your opposite hip on the seat of your chair and your back straight. Look out at the floor in front of you, not at your feet.

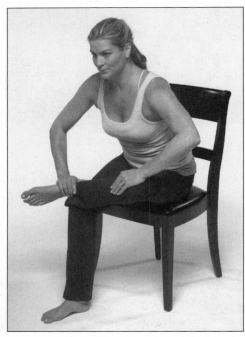

Figure 3-11:
The seated
flexibility
test for
buttocks.

3. **Make a note at what place on the clock face your knee stops moving.**

   1:00 is tight.

   2:00 is a healthy range of motion.

   3:00 is very flexible.

4. **Repeat this stretch with your right leg.**

   11:00 is tight.

   10:00 is a healthy range of motion.

   9:00 is very flexible.

Calves

Having tight calf muscles can affect not only your range of motion in your ankle but also your walking and running strides. If your calf muscles are tight and you can't get full range of motion in your ankles with this test stretch, then this lack of motion may have a negative effect on your form, in your hip, during walking and running. This imbalance may eventually lead to chronic pain or injury to your knees, hips, or even lower back.

Pay close attention to this area if you wear high heels all day. Stretching this area can help you keep your ankles, feet, and hips in balance.

To do this test stretch, follow these steps:

1. **Sit on the floor with your right leg straight out in front of you and your left leg bent so the bottom of your left foot rests against the inside thigh of your right leg.**

2. **Wrap a towel or stretching strap around the ball of your right foot and gently pull your foot toward you so your toes move toward your knee.**

    Look at Figure 3-12 if you need help. For more information about what type of strap to use, check out Chapter 2 and read the discussion on props. Also make sure to keep your back straight; don't lean forward at your hip. Try to move only your ankle and foot.

3. **Make a note on your Flexibility Self-Evaluation Worksheet at what place on the clock your toes point.**

    1:00 is tight.

    12:00 is a healthy range of motion.

    11:00 is very flexible.

4. **Repeat this stretch with your left foot.**

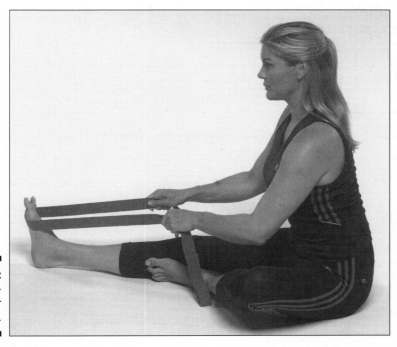

Figure 3-12: The flexibility test for your calves.

Flexibility Self-Evaluation Worksheet

To test your flexibility and record where you are now and your progress as you go along, you need to perform the test stretches in this chapter. When you finish each test stretch, record your progress in the *Clock Position* column in the evaluation sheet in Table 3-1. The description column should be used to record any information you want to note about the stretch such as level of difficulty or any discomforts you may feel.

Don't forget to make several photocopies of the worksheet in Table 3-1 so you can repeat these stretches and record your results about every six weeks. Over time you'll see how much you've improved. You'll not only feel better, but also you'll have proof that you're getting more flexible.

Table 3-1	Flexibility Self-Evaluation Worksheet		
Exercise	*Side of Body*	*Clock Position*	*Description*
Neck	Right		
	Left		
Shoulders	Right		
	Left		
Chest	N/A		
	N/A		
Trunk (four stretches)			
Seated rotation	Right		
	Left		
Standing side bend	Right		
	Left		
Seated forward bend	Right		
	Left		
Standing back extension	Right		
	Left		
Quadriceps	Right		
	Left		
Hamstrings	Right		
	Left		
Groin	Right		
	Left		
Buttocks	Right		
	Left		
Calves	Right		
	Left		

Part II
Head, Shoulders, Knees, and Toes: Targeting Specific Areas

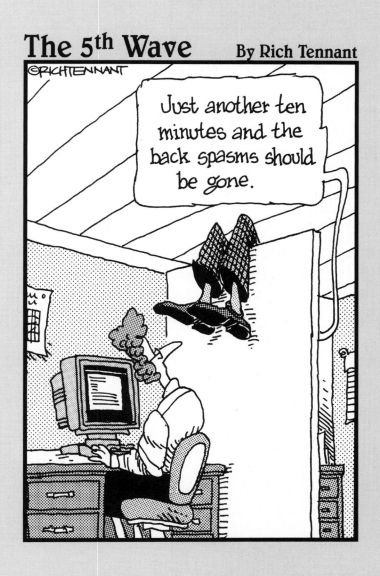

In this part . . .

No matter where you're tight, you can find a stretch that's right for you in this part because I cover stretches for every muscle in your body. I show you stretches for your neck, shoulders, chest, upper back, and arms (all parts collectively known as the upper body) in Chapter 4. Then in Chapter 5, you get a run down on some functional stretches that keep your core (your center) flexible and strong. In Chapter 6, you stretch your lower back, and finally in Chapter 7, you discover stretches for your legs, hips, and buttocks that you just can't live without!

Chapter 4

Taking It from the Top: Upper Body Stretches

Starting at the top is a good way to begin your focus for stretching the upper body because most people (including me) hold a lot of tension in the upper body. After all, the upper body is primarily made up of the neck, shoulders, and upper back. And what a powerful combination!

My dance teacher used to tell me to keep my shoulders down — I loved to bring them up around my ears whenever I got stressed. Those good old shoulders would float upward leaving me with one heck of a neckache and a tight, pinched feeling between my shoulder blades. Many people have a habit of tensing their upper body when they get stressed out, which in turn, makes the muscles in the lower body overcompensate and work harder than they really need to (leading to a backache!). And that's why this chapter is so important.

In this chapter I break down the muscles of the upper body into sections: neck, shoulders, upper back, chest, and arms. Each section gives you a few stretches that target that specific area. Pick the stretch that feels best on your body. As you get more flexible and comfortable with stretching, try some of the other stretches for variety to keep your program interesting and, dare I say, fun?

Before You Move, Contemplate Upper Body Anatomy

I always find it useful to know exactly what muscle I'm working so I can really focus on that area. To get the most out of your stretches, first locate the muscle that you're stretching by taking a look at the anatomy drawing in Figure 4-1. This picture gives you a visual reference of where the muscle is located and where it attaches so you can stretch it more effectively. Having this visual helps you achieve a mind/body connection. By this, I mean that your mind is aware of what your body is doing. When you perform a stretch, picture the muscle from the drawing in your mind and feel it in your body.

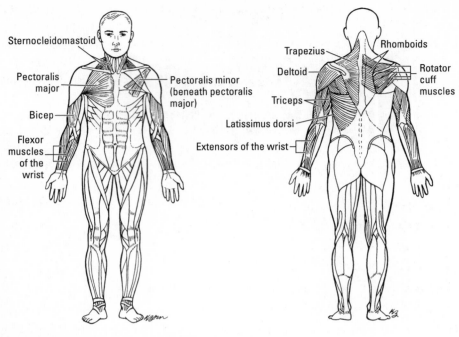

Sternocleidomastoid

Pectoralis major

Bicep

Flexor muscles of the wrist

Pectoralis minor (beneath pectoralis major)

Trapezius

Rhomboids

Deltoid

Rotator cuff muscles

Triceps

Latissimus dorsi

Extensors of the wrist

Figure 4-1:
Full body anatomy drawing with neck and shoulders highlighted (front and back).

Note: Sternocleidomastoid muscle has 2 parts as indicated.

What a Pain in the Neck! Stretches to Keep Your Head Held High

For most people, the neck is a lightning rod for stress. Traffic, job issues, cranky children — it's amazing that the tension created by frustrations such as these are stored in that tiny little area above your shoulders and below your head. The movement of the head and neck is very complex and involves many muscles working together. To keep it simple, focus on four of those muscles: Upper trapezius (truh-*pee*-zee-uhs), sternocleidomastoid (stur-noh-klahy-duh-*mas*-toid), scalenes (skey-*leens*), and levator scapula (li-*vey*-ter *skap*-yuh-luh). These are the muscles that, when not taken care of, literally become a pain in the neck.

Regularly stretching the muscles of your neck can reduce pain and tightness that if left unchecked can lead to headaches, chronic stiffness, limited range of motion, and even carpal tunnel syndrome. The stretches in this section may even prevent pain altogether.

Lateral head tilt

The lateral head tilt stretches the muscles that run along the sides of your neck: anterior, middle, and posterior scalenes. These muscles attach to the upper rib cage, so to get an effective stretch, you have to anchor your shoulder blades down as you tilt your head to the side.

To do this stretch, follow these steps:

1. **Inhale as you lift your shoulders up to your ears with your arms straight down at your sides.**

2. **Exhale and lower your shoulders and anchor your shoulder blades in place to provide a firm foundation for the stretch.**

3. **Tilt your head to the left side, moving your left ear toward your left shoulder (see Figure 4-2), being very careful not to lift your right shoulder.**

Imagine that you're holding a very heavy book in your hand as you tilt your head to the opposite side. This thought may help you keep your right shoulder down and allow you to feel the stretch more.

4. **Hold the stretch for two or three deep breaths and then lift your head back to center.**

5. **Inhale as you lift your shoulders again; exhale as you lower your shoulders.**

6. **Repeat the stretch on the right side.**

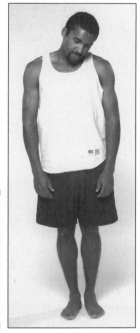

Figure 4-2:
The lateral head tilt includes the shoulder shrug and side neck stretch.

A few do's and don'ts for this stretch:

✔ Do be aware of your muscles in your upper back holding your shoulder down.

✔ Do breathe as you hold the stretch.

✔ Do sit or stand up tall as you hold the stretch.

✔ Don't tilt from your waist.

✔ Don't let your opposite shoulder lift as you tilt your head.

Neck rotation with tilt

Doing this stretch can be effective for immediate pain control and also, if done consistently, can actually help prevent pain in the future because it targets the trapezius — the main culprit in stress headaches!

This stretch can be done sitting or standing, but just remember that to effectively stretch this area you must anchor your shoulder blades or keep them still to provide a solid foundation for the stretch.

To do this stretch, follow these steps:

1. **Find a stable, flat chair that you can sit comfortably in and position yourself in an upright, military-type posture.**

2. **Slowly rotate your head to the right approximately 45 degrees and slowly lean forward and drop your head slightly (see Figure 4-3).**

   You should begin to feel tension build lightly over the right shoulder and neck.

3. **Hold this position, maintaining the light to medium stretch for at least one _full_ minute.**

4. **Repeat on the other side by simply reversing the above instructions.**

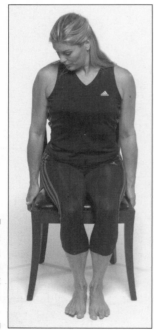

Figure 4-3:
The neck rotation with tilt is great for relieving tension.

A few do's and don'ts for this stretch:

- ✔ Do breathe as you hold the stretch.
- ✔ Do hold your shoulders down while you tilt your head to the side.
- ✔ Do sit up or stand up tall as you hold the stretch.
- ✔ Don't let your shoulders round forward as you drop your head.
- ✔ Don't yank or force the stretch.

Neck rotation

The primary muscle that turns your head side to side is your sternocleidomastoid. No, you don't have to know how to spell it, but take a look at Figure 4-1 to see where it's located. It's important to keep flexibility in this area because many of the movements in life require you to turn your head. Every time you look over your shoulder, you use this muscle.

Perform the following steps for this exercise:

1. **Inhale and make sure that your shoulders are down, chest is lifted, and abdominals are in.**

2. **As you exhale, slowly turn your head to the right (see Figure 4-4).**

3. **Find a focal point to stare at and hold this position for five seconds.**

4. **Inhale and release back to center.**

5. **As you exhale, turn your head again in the same direction and find another focal point a little farther than the first.**

6. **Hold this stretch for five seconds and release back to center.**

7. **Repeat the series, looking in the other direction.**

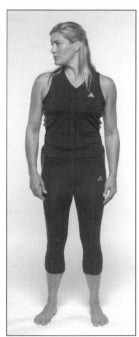

Figure 4-4: The neck rotation.

A few do's and don'ts for this stretch:

✔ Do breathe as you hold the stretch.

✔ Do anchor your shoulders so they face forward. You don't want your shoulders to move as you turn your head.

✔ Do sit up or stand up tall as you hold the stretch.

✔ Don't yank or force the stretch or you'll do more harm than good; because these muscles work so hard all day holding your head up, they're delicately balanced and easily injured.

Relieving headaches

Statistics show that over 90 percent of people have a headache at some time in their life, which, amazingly, means that a lucky 10 percent of people never have a headache. But a headache can happen at any time, anywhere, and can definitely ruin your day. And even though headaches are common, most people don't have any idea where a headache comes from.

Tension headaches are by far the most common form of headaches and can be due to stress, which causes you to clench or strain the muscles of your face, neck, jaw, and/or shoulders. When these muscles are tight they can compress the nerves that lead to your scalp, causing a tight, squeezing sensation in your head. Fatigue, lack of sleep, or even sleep disorders can also result in this type of headache.

Posture also plays a key role in many tension headaches. Many of the positions we habitually put ourselves in tighten neck and back muscles. Try to avoid constantly tilting your head to one side (a problem for frequent phone users). Be aware of your posture as you sit at your desk, drive your car, stand in line at the grocery store, or carry a bag or purse.

Migraines are generally less common headaches but more severe. Although stress can be a major trigger for migraine headache, migraines and cluster headaches are regarded as primarily vascular in nature, and not necessarily the result of muscle tightness. What triggers a migraine headache in one person may have no effect in someone else, including hormone fluctuations, smoking, chocolate, and even the weather.

When it comes to relieving the pain of occasional tension headaches, thousands of people turn to over-the-counter drugs such as aspirin, acetaminophen, or ibuprofen, which can be very effective. In addition, some proven-effective natural remedies include

- Ice packs
- A warm shower or bath
- Massaging the neck and shoulders
- Aerobic exercise (to promote the release of endorphins and relax tight muscles)
- Eating regularly
- Sex
- A glass of wine

Treatment for recurrent tension headaches, however, is another story. A frequently throbbing head is your body's way of telling you that something significant is out of balance in your life. Stress is an unavoidable part of modern life, but by far the best course of action to combat stress-related tension headaches is prevention. Although such natural remedies as a visit to a chiropractor, acupressure, acupuncture, and even hypnosis can help with recurring tension headaches, several well-regarded studies have concluded that stress management skills and relaxation training can reduce chronic headache for 50 to 70 percent of patients. Techniques such as deep breathing, meditation, and most important of all, stretching, can trigger the relaxation response, which can lower blood pressure, reduce pulse rates, and release muscle tension. Regular stretching keeps you calm and flexible, and it can help reduce headache frequency and intensity.

The Hot Seat for Tension: Getting Your Shoulders to Chill Out

The main focus when stretching the shoulder is the deltoid muscle — the muscle that runs over the outside of your shoulder. When you think about the deltoid, remember that it's really three muscles in one: front, middle, and back (refer to Figure 4-1). So to truly stretch your shoulder, you need to stretch all three parts of the deltoid. (Don't worry; I show you how in the following sections.)

In addition to the deltoid muscle, a collection of small but extremely important muscles and tendons deep within the shoulder joint is called the *rotator cuff*. Because a strong and flexible rotator cuff is essential for an effective throwing motion, keeping this area in tiptop shape is the key point for baseball pitchers. Check out the following stretches to help you keep alive your dream of having a major league pitching career (or perhaps just to play catch with your grandkids without pain).

Middle of shoulder stretch

If you want to know what your deltoid muscle does, just lift your arm in any direction. Try moving your arm forward or back, overhead, in a circular motion, or just straight up and down. None of these movements is possible without your deltoid doing most of the work. Because your deltoids are so active and used in almost every movement that involves your arms, they're contracted constantly throughout your day. This constant tension creates tightness in your shoulders, which is all the more reason to stretch this area daily.

The following stretch is specifically for the middle part of your deltoid. This stretch can be done sitting, standing, or lying down. Just make sure to maintain good posture so you feel the full effectiveness of the stretch.

To do this stretch, follow these steps:

1. **Sit up straight with your feet flat on the floor and your abdominals lifted.**

2. **Lift your right arm across your chest and hook the left arm under your right arm (see Figure 4-5a).**

   If your shoulders are extremely stiff or tight and you find it difficult to hook your arm underneath your other arm, try the stretch lying on your back. Just drape your arm across your body and let gravity do the work. You may find it more comfortable.

3. **Now, gently lower your right shoulder so it's even with your left shoulder (see Figure 4-5b).**

4. **Inhale and as you exhale use your left arm to gently pull your right arm across your body.**

5. **Hold the stretch for 30 seconds or four to five slow, deep breaths.**

6. **Repeat the stretch with the left arm.**

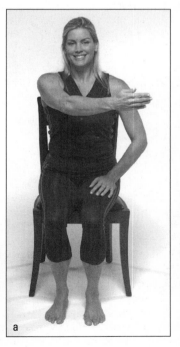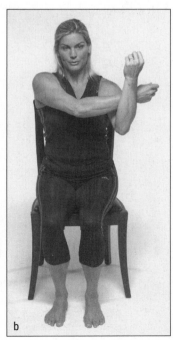

Figure 4-5:
Middle of shoulder stretch.

a

b

A few do's and don'ts for this stretch:

- ✔ Do breathe as you hold the stretch.
- ✔ Do progress through the stretch gradually.
- ✔ Do sit up or stand up tall as you hold the stretch.
- ✔ Don't let your shoulder lift or kink your neck.
- ✔ Don't pull too forcefully.

Back of shoulder stretch

This stretch is specifically for the back part of your deltoid and can be performed either sitting or standing. Just remember to keep your core stable and supported.

To do this stretch, follow these steps:

1. **Sit or stand up straight with your feet flat on the floor and contract your abdominals.**
2. **Place your right arm straight out in front of you so it's level with your chest.**
3. **Bend your elbow so your hand moves upward and is level with your chin.**
4. **Bring your left arm under your right and intertwine your forearms with your palms facing out (see Figure 4-6a).**

   Don't worry if you can't get your arms completely intertwined. Just cross your arms at your elbows and lift. As you get more flexible, you may notice a greater range of motion.
5. **Inhale and as you exhale, lift both elbows about an inch (see Figure 4-6b).**
6. **Hold for 30 seconds or four to five slow, deep breaths.**
7. **Repeat this stretch with your right arm under your left.**

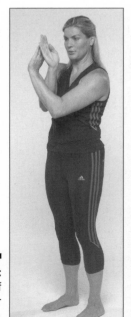
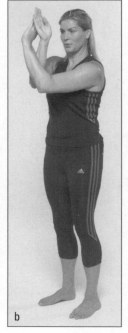

Figure 4-6: Back of shoulder stretch.

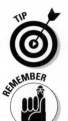

Don't worry if you can't get your arms completely intertwined. Just cross your arms at your elbows and lift. As you get more flexible, you may notice a greater range of motion.

A few do's and don'ts for this stretch:

- ✔ Do breathe as you hold the stretch.
- ✔ Do progress through the stretch gradually.
- ✔ Do sit up tall as you hold the stretch.
- ✔ Don't let your shoulder lift and don't kink your neck.

Shoulder rotation stretch

You'll feel this stretch all around your shoulders because it targets the smaller, deeper muscles known as your rotator cuff and the front part of your deltoid known as the anterior deltoid. You need a stretching strap (see Chapter 2 for more details about straps) or towel for this stretch.

To do this stretch, follow these steps:

1. **Stand up very tall with your feet about hip-width apart.**

2. **Grab each end of your towel or strap with your palms down and resting in front of your thighs (see Figure 4-7a).**

3. **Straighten your arms and inhale as you raise your arms overhead (see Figure 4-7b).**

4. **Exhale and take your arms farther behind your head without arching your back.**

5. **Hold the stretch for 30 seconds or for four to five slow, deep breaths.**

Figure 4-7: Shoulder rotation stretch.

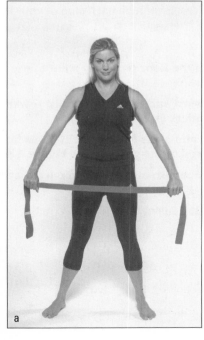

a

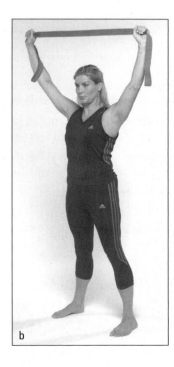

b

If you're having trouble keeping your back straight, check out the lying arm circles stretch from Chapter 8. That exercise may help remind your body of how to keep your core stable as you move your shoulders.

A few do's and don'ts for this stretch:

✔ Do keep your arms symmetrical as you hold the stretch.

✔ Do progress through the stretch gradually and slowly.

✔ Do stand up tall as you hold the stretch.

✔ Don't twist to either side.

✔ Don't bounce or force the stretch.

Stretches for Carrying Someone on Your Lats

The main muscles in your upper back are the *latissimus dorsi* (pronounced luh-*tis*-uh-muhs *dawr*-sahy and commonly known as the *lats, trapezius,* or *traps*) and the rhomboids, which unfortunately don't have a catchy nickname. These muscles play an important role in stabilizing your spine, moving your arms, and maintaining good posture. The following upper back stretches involve all these muscles on both sides of the body.

Lat stretch on all fours

This position is a great stretch for your latissimus dorsi — the largest muscle in your back. Even though this muscle is located on your back, it attaches to your arm; therefore, you need to reach with your arms to fully stretch this muscle. Also, your lats attach to your lower back, so tightness in this muscle can create pain and imbalance in your lower back. As you reach in this stretch, you feel your muscles stretch on each side of your back.

When doing this stretch, follow these steps:

1. **Begin with your knees and your hands on the floor (you may want to use an exercise mat to cushion your hands and knees).**

2. **Exhale and reach your arms straight forward and lower your chest toward the floor, keeping your hips higher than your shoulders (see Figure 4-8a).**

3. **Inhale, exhale, and move your shoulders and arms toward the right as far as you can reach and still keep your hips anchored to the ground (see Figure 4-8b).**

4. **Hold for 30 seconds or four to five slow, deep breaths and then move back to center position.**

5. **Repeat the same stretch but reach to the left instead.**

A few do's and don'ts for this stretch:

✔ Do feel a slight arch in your back.

✔ Do press your chest toward the floor and keep your hips high.

✔ Do progress through the stretch gradually and slowly.

> ✔ Don't round your back.
> ✔ Don't move your hips.

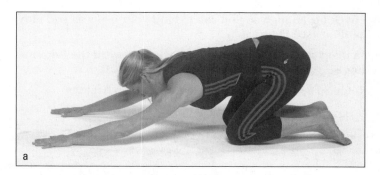

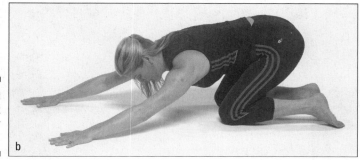

Figure 4-8:
Upper back
stretch for
your lats.

Supported upper back stretch

What I like about the supported upper back stretch is that you don't have to get down on the floor to do it. It's easy to do at the gym, at home, or outdoors. Just find a sturdy support that is about hip height. Be creative — if you're outdoors, use the back of a park bench or even a tree. If you're at the gym, you probably can find a ballet barre, a ledge, or a railing. And if you're at home, use the kitchen counter or table.

Modify the supported upper back stretch

Try out the following tips to modify the supported upper back stretch (shown in Figure 4-9):

✔ If you have tight hamstrings and feel pain in the back of your thighs, bend your knees slightly during the stretch. This adaptation helps relieve the tension in the back of your thighs so you can focus on stretching your upper back. After you finish this stretch you may want to read Chapter 7, where I give you many stretches for your unhappy hamstrings.

To make this a more warm-up type stretch, try doing this stretch in a more rhythmic movement of slightly arching and rounding your back, moving with each breath.

✔ As you hold the stretch, try dropping one shoulder a little lower than the other. This version can help deepen the stretch on the side of your back with the lowered shoulder.

To do this stretch, follow these steps:

1. **Stand with your feet about hip-width apart and place your hands on a sturdy surface for support.**

2. **Move your feet back far enough so you can extend your arms as you move your chest toward the floor (see Figure 4-9).**

3. **Exhale and get a deep stretch by pressing your chest toward the floor and your hips toward the ceiling so you have a slight arch in your back.**

4. **Hold the stretch for 30 seconds or four to five slow, deep breaths.**

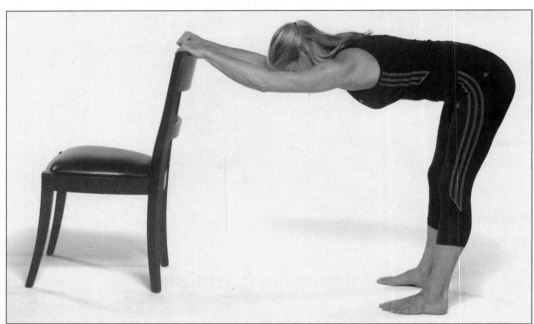

Figure 4-9:
Supported
upper back
stretch.

A few do's and don'ts for this stretch:

✔ Do keep your neck in line with the rest of your spine.

✔ Do use your breath to relax into the stretch.

✔ Don't drop your chin to your chest.

✔ Don't round your spine.

Seated upper back stretch

This stretch targets the smaller muscles in your upper back — specifically the rhomboids — and you should feel this stretch between your shoulder blades. It's important to keep this muscle group strong and flexible because the rhomboids play an important role in good posture.

Ironically, for many people, their rhomboids are weak and overstretched. If you find that your shoulders roll forward when you stand or sit, you probably need to focus on strengthening these upper back muscles. To find out more about strengthening this area, consult a private trainer or a book on weight training such as *Weight Training For Dummies,* 3rd Edition, by Shirley Archer (Wiley).

To do this stretch, follow these steps:

1. **Sit on the floor with your knees slightly bent and your arms crossed behind your knees (see Figure 4-10a).**

2. **Inhale as you lean forward, letting your chest rest on your thighs.**

3. **As you exhale, round your back and pull away from your knees, but be sure that your arms are locked under your knees (see Figure 4-10b).**

4. **Hold this position for 30 seconds or four to five slow, deep breaths.**

Figure 4-10:
Seated
upper back
stretch.

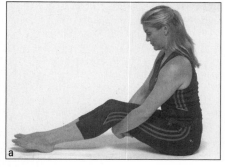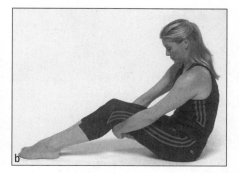

A few do's and don'ts for this stretch:

✔ Do feel your shoulder blades move away from each other.

✔ Do tilt your pelvis under.

✔ Don't tense up your shoulders.

✔ Don't hold your breath.

Both Sexes, Take Care! The Kneeling Chest Stretch

The official names for the muscles of your chest are *pectoralis major* and *pectoralis minor* — more commonly known as the *pecs* (pectoralis is pronounced pek-tuh-*ral*-is). Whether you exercise regularly or you're a perfect couch potato, if you don't stretch these muscles regularly, they can tighten and shorten, which cause your shoulders to round forward.

Most people already have weak upper back muscles, and this constant pulling from tight pecs weakens your back muscles even further, creating even more of an imbalance between your chest and upper back muscles. The end result is rounded shoulders and poor posture (and your mother shouting at you to stop slouching!).

The following stretch is designed to help increase the range of motion in your shoulders by lengthening and stretching the pectoralis major. To do this stretch, follow these steps:

1. **Kneel on a carpeted floor or mat with your forearms crossed and resting on the seat of a sturdy chair (see Figure 4-11a).**

2. **Breathe in and as you exhale let your head and chest sink below the chair seat (see Figure 4-11b).**

3. **Hold the stretch for 30 seconds and feel your shoulders and upper chest stretch, while you use deep breathing to help you sink gradually deeper into the stretch.**

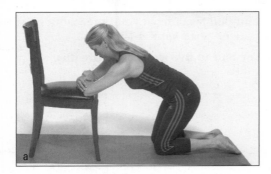

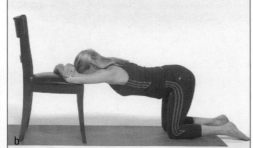

Figure 4-11: Kneeling chest stretch.

A few do's and don'ts for this stretch:

✔ Do start the stretch in the comfort zone and gradually progress into a deep stretch.

✔ Do avoid arching or rounding your back.

✔ Don't allow your pelvis to tilt back or tuck under.

Making Wiggly Muscles Firm: Stretches for the Dreaded Upper Arm

If you're a woman of a certain age, you may have been led to believe that, like death and taxes, flabby upper arms are inevitable at some point. Well, I'm here to tell you that doesn't have to be the case. Upper arm development and definition are a big goal for *both* men and women. Men love to show off their "guns" and women are constantly looking for the solution for their flabby upper arms. With the focus on toning this area, remember it's just as important to stretch and lengthen these muscles too. By lengthening the muscles on the front and back of the upper arm, stretching can aid in bringing firmness and definition to this area by allowing the muscles to respond more effectively to toning exercises.

Biceps and triceps are the two main muscles of your upper arm. The biceps (your "guns") are in the front of your upper arm. Contracting your biceps muscles bends your elbow. Your triceps are smaller and a little better hidden in the back of your upper arm. Contracting your triceps straightens your elbow. With that in mind, to stretch your biceps you need to straighten your elbow and to stretch your triceps you need to bend your elbow.

Back of the arms stretch

It's no secret that doing push-ups will work the muscles of your chest. But did you know that when you do a push-up it also works your triceps? That's because your triceps help your chest muscles when you push something away.

This traditional stretch for the back of your upper arm can be done sitting or standing. Another good triceps stretch is patting yourself on the back when you're finished!

To do this stretch, follow these steps:

1. **Raise one arm overhead and bend your arm at the elbow so your fingers are reaching down your spine and your elbow is pointing upward.**

2. **Place your other hand on your raised elbow and as you exhale gently press your elbow back so your fingers reach farther down your spine (see Figure 4-12).**

   If reaching overhead is awkward or uncomfortable, try the stretch with your raised elbow against a wall, and use the wall to apply the pressure to your elbow.

3. **Hold the stretch for 30 seconds or four to five slow, deep breaths.**

4. **Repeat this stretch with your other arm.**

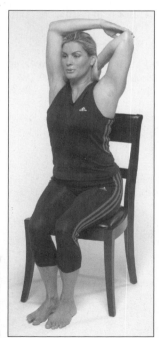

Figure 4-12:
Back of
the arms
stretch.

A few do's and don'ts for this stretch:

- ✔ Do keep your eyes looking forward.
- ✔ Do keep your back straight and deepen the stretch by moving your elbow back, not by moving your rib cage forward.
- ✔ Do try to walk your finger tips farther down your back.
- ✔ Don't arch your back.
- ✔ Don't force or bounce the stretch.

Triceps stretch with towel or strap

When you're doing the triceps stretch, remember to maintain good posture throughout the exercise. You may sit or stand during this stretch, and you need a towel, so go grab one now. Using the towel helps people who are very tight in the shoulders because the towel allows you to focus on your triceps without feeling discomfort in your shoulders.

To do this stretch, follow these steps:

1. **Place your towel or strap in your left hand and lift it over your shoulder.**
2. **With your right hand, reach behind your back and grab the other end of the towel (see Figure 4-13).**
3. **Inhale and as you exhale, gently pull down on the towel with your right hand.**
4. **With each exhale try to increase the stretch by pulling down on the towel a little more with your right hand.**
5. **Hold the stretch for 30 seconds or four to five slow, deep breaths.**
6. **Repeat this stretch with your right arm.**

You can get a stretch in your shoulder at the same time if you walk your lower hand up the towel as you gently pull down on the towel, as if you were trying to get your two hands to touch.

A few do's and don'ts for this stretch:

- ✔ Do keep your back straight and your abdominals in.
- ✔ Do relax as you hold the stretch.
- ✔ Do keep your eyes forward and your shoulder blades down.
- ✔ Don't hold your breath.
- ✔ Don't bounce the stretch or yank on the towel too forcefully.
- ✔ Don't tuck your chin down to your chest.

Standing biceps stretch

This upper arm stretch is great for your biceps because you don't need props. No need to wait until after your workout to perform this stretch. Try doing it right after you complete your biceps curls during your upper body workout.

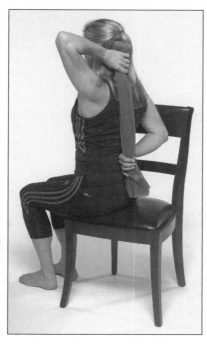

Figure 4-13:
Triceps
stretch using
a towel
or strap.

To do this stretch, follow these steps:

1. **Stand up tall with your feet shoulder-width apart and your arms extended to the side, palms facing forward — about shoulder height (see Figure 4-14a).**

2. **Inhale and as you exhale rotate your thumbs downward and back (see Figure 4-14b).**

3. **Hold the stretch for 30 seconds and release.**

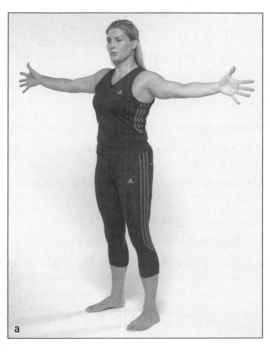
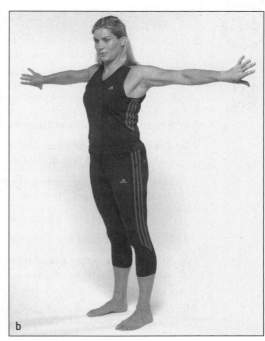

Figure 4-14:
Standing
biceps
stretch.

A few do's and don'ts for this stretch:

- Do breathe through the entire stretch.
- Do stay relaxed.
- Do keep your shoulders down and chest lifted.
- Do look forward through the entire stretch.
- Don't let your shoulders round.
- Don't drop your head forward.

Helping You Hold Your Extra-Large Handbag: Wrist and Forearm Stretches

People who work with their hands (including people who work on a computer a lot) know all about the danger of strain or overuse. Many office workers, in fact, suffer from chronic hand pain and can even have *carpal tunnel syndrome,* which is a painful condition that occurs when a key nerve that runs from your forearm to your hand gets squeezed or pinched.

The repetitive motion of racquet sports can also create tension in the wrists and forearms. Taking a few minutes a day to stretch your wrists may be just what you need to prevent future chronic pain in your hands and wrists. The following stretches can be done any time and any place, and especially at work whenever you feel you need a break.

Wrist stretch on hands and knees

Keeping the muscles of the wrists and forearms flexible is extremely important in the prevention of repetitive motion injuries such as tennis elbow or carpal tunnel syndrome. If these areas are tight, the muscles and tendons can be forced beyond their natural range of movement. If you have or think you may have carpal tunnel syndrome, you may want to skip this stretch.

To do this stretch, follow these steps:

1. **Kneel on all fours with most of your weight on your knees.**

2. **Turn the wrist of your left hand so your fingers point toward your knees and your palm is toward the floor (see Figure 4-15a).**

3. **Inhale and as you exhale gently lower the palm of your hand to the floor as you shift your hips toward your heels.**

   You should feel the stretch in the palm of your hand and forearm.

4. **Hold the stretch for 30 seconds or four to five slow, deep breaths.**

5. **Release the stretch and lift your left hand off the floor and turn your wrist so the back of your hand is now on the floor with your fingers toward your knees (see Figure 4-15b).**

6. **Inhale and as you exhale gently move your wrist toward the floor and your hips toward your heels.**

7. Hold for 30 seconds or four to five slow, deep breaths.

8. Repeat these two stretches on your other wrist.

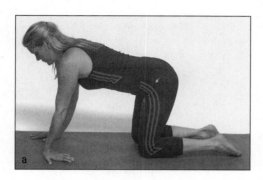

Figure 4-15:
Wrist
stretch on
hands and
knees.

A few do's and don'ts for this stretch:

✔ Do keep your shoulder blades down and your body weight shifting toward your heels.

✔ Don't put all your weight on the wrist that you're stretching.

✔ Don't bounce in the stretch.

Standing open-arm wrist stretch

You'll feel this stretch in your forearms, wrists, and the palms of your hands. It is very subtle, so you need to focus to really feel the stretch. Also, keep in mind that you can do this stretch standing or sitting, whichever is more comfortable for you. Just remember that if you round your shoulders forward, you probably won't feel the full effect of the stretch — so keep those shoulders back.

To do this stretch, follow these steps:

1. Stand tall with your back straight and your chest lifted.

2. Extend your arms to the side — no higher than shoulder height — with palms facing forward (see Figure 4-16a).

3. Open your hands as wide as you can with your fingers reaching long and apart.

4. Bend your wrists toward the back wall, and then move your arms back an inch or two (see Figure 4-16b).

5. Hold the stretch for 30 seconds or four to five slow, deep breaths.

Keep reminding yourself to keep your hands wide open; otherwise, your hands start to relax and the stretch isn't as effective.

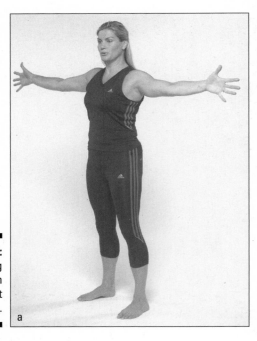 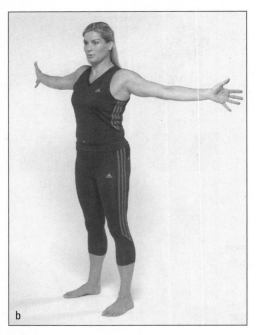

Figure 4-16:
Standing
open-arm
wrist
stretch.

a

b

A few do's and don'ts for this stretch:

- ✔ Do keep your shoulder blades down.
- ✔ Do keep your arms extended.
- ✔ Don't bend your elbows.
- ✔ Don't slouch.

Chapter 5

Centering on the Core: Stretches for Your Middle

....

In This Chapter

▶ Getting familiar with the muscles of your core

▶ Discovering what core muscles do

▶ Creating some functional stretches for your core

▶ Discovering the best static and dynamic stretches for your core

....

Your core is made up of the muscles of your back, abs, hips, and even your chest (see Figure 5-1). Because these core muscles all work together to support your spine, they're the foundation of all movement in your body for not only sports but also for daily life. Whether you play tennis or just reach for something on the top shelf in your kitchen, the movement actually begins with your core muscles, not with your arms. All your muscles are connected to each other, so it seems logical that they have an effect on each other. In other words, being tight in one area or muscle can limit your movement and cause you to overcompensate with other muscles. (Remember that old song: "*Your foot bone's connected to your ankle bone; your ankle bone's connected to your shin bone . . .* "? That's the principle here.) This whole process can be the start of improper movement patterns, which may lead to injuries and painful complications. It's because of this threat of injury that core training has become so popular. But it's not enough just to strengthen these muscles; you need to lengthen them as well to maintain a healthy range of motion.

All the stretches in this chapter are what I call *integrated stretches,* meaning you stretch several muscles at the same time. The first series of stretches are functional stretches, which mimic normal activities. These exercises are also known as *dynamic, active stretches* (discussed in more detail in Chapter 1). The second series of stretches are called *static stretches* and target the abdominals, back, and waist to help improve range of motion. The combination of these stretches helps create a strong and flexible core.

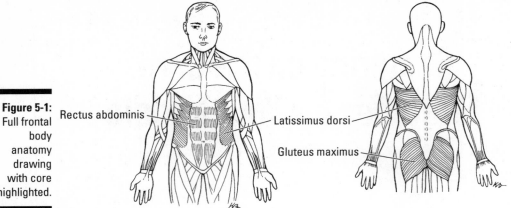

Figure 5-1:
Full frontal
body
anatomy
drawing
with core
highlighted.

Rectus abdominis

Latissimus dorsi

Gluteus maximus

Active Stretches as Part of the Day-to-Day

Functional stretches mimic life. Reaching, twisting, and bending are everyday movements, which require many muscles to work together at the same time. These stretches are called *active, dynamic stretches* in which you move through the stretch and do several repetitions, but you don't necessarily have to hold the stretch for the full 30 seconds.

A great additional benefit of these functional core stretches is that you actually *strengthen* your muscles as you stretch and lengthen them. A fitness daily double!

Step back with overhead reach

This abdominal stretch is for the muscles that run along the front of your torso. Feel this stretch in your hip flexor, abdominals, and chest. A couple of important points to focus on during this stretch include the following:

✔ To really feel a deeper stretch in your hip flexor, tuck your pelvis under as you step back.

✔ Think of your spine as lengthening, not shortening, so the focus is on the front of your torso and not your lower back.

To do this stretch, follow these steps:

1. **Stand tall with your feet together, your abdominals and chest lifted, your shoulders back, and your shoulder blades down (see Figure 5-2a).**

2. **Inhale and as you exhale, lunge back with your left leg and reach your left arm over your head (see Figure 5-2b).**

3. **Hold this position for three deep breaths.**

4. **Inhale and bring your foot and arm back to starting position.**

5. **Repeat this exercise with your right leg and arm.**

6. **Repeat this stretch for six to eight repetitions, alternating sides (as in Step 5).**

   When you feel you're ready to add a repetition or two, try doing two sets of six to eight repetitions.

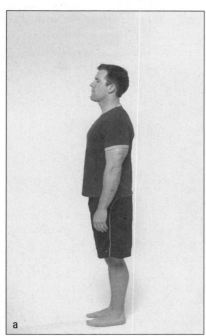
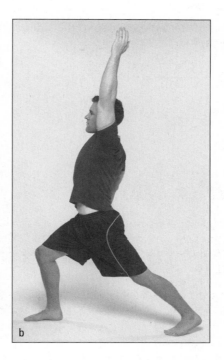

Figure 5-2:
Step back
lunge with
overhead
reach.

a

b

A few do's and don'ts for this stretch:

- ✔ Do keep your spine long, even as you reach up and back down.
- ✔ Do keep the motion slow and fluid and use your abdominals to slow that motion down.
- ✔ Do use your upper back muscles to keep your shoulder blade down as you reach overhead.
- ✔ Don't compress your lower back as you reach up.
- ✔ Don't twist or reach to the side.

Alternating side reach with hip stretch

This reach-and-stretch exercise is for the muscles that run along the outside of your hip, and the movements help your abdominals and your back. This stretch is a great daily stretch to keep you sitting tall and exercise good posture.

Perform this stretch by following the steps below:

1. **Stand up tall with your feet together, your abdominals and chest lifted, your shoulders back, and your shoulder blades down (see Figure 5-3a).**

2. **Inhale and as you exhale, step out to the side with your right leg (side lunge), reaching your right arm overhead in the opposite direction (see Figure 5-3b).**

   The farther out you step to the side, the more you feel a stretch in your inner thigh, too.

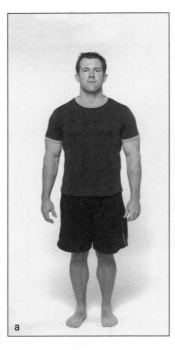 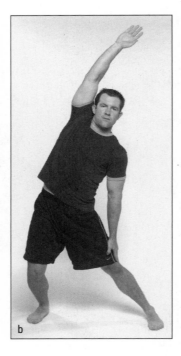

Figure 5-3:
Side reach with hip stretch.

a

b

3. **Hold the stretch for one deep breath.**

4. **Inhale and bring your body back to the starting position.**

5. **Repeat the steps on the left side.**

6. **Repeat this stretch for six to eight repetitions, alternating sides (as in Step 5).**

   When you feel you're ready to add a repetition or two, try doing two sets of six to eight repetitions.

A few do's and don'ts for this stretch:

- ✔ Do keep your stationary leg straight so you feel the stretch in your inner thigh.
- ✔ Don't twist or rotate your hips.
- ✔ Don't bend forward as you lunge to the side.

The chop

The chop, so named because of its similar move as in chopping wood, is the king of all functional stretches because it stretches your buttocks, back, abs, and chest all at the same time. To do this stretch, follow these steps:

1. **Stand up tall with your feet hip-width apart and your arms at your sides.**

2. **Bend your knees and pivot on your left big toe as you lift your left heel.**

   Your right foot remains on the ground and should be facing forward (see Figure 5-4a).

3. **Twist your hips to the right and reach both of your arms down and behind you.**

4. **Hold the position for one deep breath.**

5. **Come back to center and continue to turn your hips as you reach both arms overhead to the left (see Figure 5-4b).**

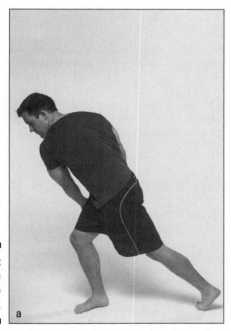 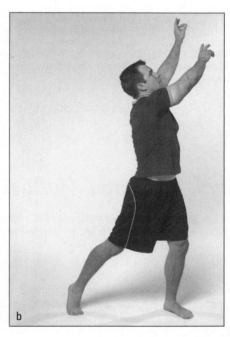

Figure 5-4: An example of how to do the chop.

a

b

6. **Hold this position for one deep breath.**

   You should feel the stretch in your right hip flexor, obliques, and chest.

7. **Repeat the stretch from right to left for six to eight repetitions and then work your way up to two sets of eight repetitions as you feel more comfortable.**

To protect your back and spine, your hips should move with you and not remain forward throughout the moves.

A few do's and don'ts for this stretch:

✔ Do inhale as you reach up and exhale as you bring your arms back down.

✔ Do lengthen your spine throughout the movement.

✔ Do hold your abdominals tight to protect your back.

✔ Don't arch or compress your lower back.

✔ Don't let your knees bow in or collapse inward.

✔ Don't swing or create too much momentum; keep the movement fluid and under control.

Static Stretches for Your Core

The next three exercises are static stretches that help increase your range of motion throughout your core. Stretching the abdominals protects the back and prevents injury and vice versa.

With static stretches for your core (and for any other stretch for that matter), take the time to slow down and focus on holding the stretch because it strengthens the muscles you're working.

Pilates is a great example of static stretching because it involves holding a series of movements as you slow down and focus your breathing on each exercise. Check out *Pilates For Dummies* by Ellie Herman (Wiley) for some great workouts with static stretches.

Back extension (for your abdominals — go figure)

You see people every day who walk through life with rounded backs. You may even have this issue yourself. The back extension stretch is here to help you! This stretch is technically for the abdominals, but it's also great for the back muscles because it moves your spine in the opposite direction, giving the muscles a workout and increasing the mobility of your spine.

To do this stretch, follow these steps:

1. **Lie on your belly and prop yourself up with your elbows.**

   Your elbows should be directly under your shoulders. Make sure that you lift yourself up out of your shoulders so that you aren't sinking into your shoulder blades.

2. **Inhale and as you exhale, lengthen your spine and lift your chest as if you were going to move forward (see Figure 5-5).**

   While performing this stretch, imagine that you're trying to move forward but your elbows and hips are glued to the floor and the space between each vertebra is increasing, lengthening your spine.

3. **Hold the stretch for 30 seconds or four to five slow, deep breaths.**

   You should feel this stretch in your abdominals.

4. **Repeat the stretch for six to eight repetitions or whatever feels most comfortable to you.**

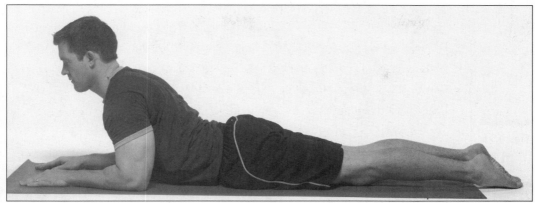

Figure 5-5:
The back extension that stretches the abdominals.

A few do's and don'ts for this stretch:

  ✔ Do keep your neck long and in line with the rest of your spine.

  ✔ Do pull your belly in toward your spine.

  ✔ Don't compress your lower back.

  ✔ Don't lift your chest toward the ceiling; think of your chest moving forward and up.

Lying spinal rotation

The lying spinal rotation is a good stretch to do when you want to stretch several muscles at once. In this stretch, you feel your back, oblique, neck, and chest muscles all stretch at the same time.

This stretch may be a bit uncomfortable at first, so always begin the stretch in your comfort zone for the first 10 to 15 seconds of the stretch, and then gradually increase the resistance of the stretch for the remainder. Never stretch beyond your pain threshold. Beginning slowly gives your muscles a chance to release and loosen up before you try to deepen the stretch.

If at any time during this stretch you feel stress and tightness in your back instead of relaxation and lengthening, try keeping both knees bent or placing a block or folded towel under your knee.

This stretch involves the following steps:

  1. **Lie on your back with both legs extended and both arms extended out from your sides.**

  2. **Inhale and raise your left knee to your chest; slowly cross your knee over your body to the right (see Figure 5-6).**

  3. **Turn your head to the left or opposite direction as you relax into the stretch.**

     Make sure to keep both arms and shoulder blades on the floor during this stretch.

  4. **Hold the stretch for 30 seconds; release the stretch, and repeat on the other side.**

This stretch can also stretch your neck, so to do this, look toward your extended arm as you hold the stretch.

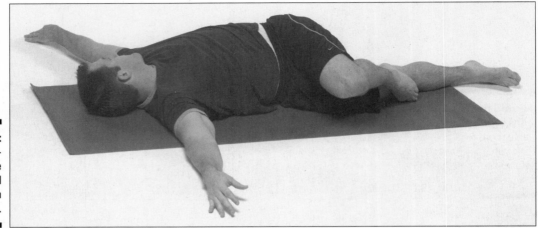

Figure 5-6:
How to perform the lying spinal rotation stretch.

A few do's and don'ts for this stretch:

- Do breathe regularly as you hold the stretch.
- Do progress through the stretch gradually.
- Don't arch your back.
- Don't force your knee to the floor; it's better to keep your shoulder blades on the floor than to get your knee to touch the floor.

Spinal rotation for back and buttocks

A traditional stretch exists to stretch your buttocks, but by adding a spinal rotation to this buttocks stretch, you can stretch your back and buttocks at the same time. The two-in-one stretch can save you time and stretch your muscles more functionally.

A normal function of your daily routine — like bending down and reaching across to pick something up — requires the muscles of your hip to stretch at the same time as the lats on the other side of your back. Stretching this area keeps you flexible.

To do this stretch, follow these steps:

1. **Stand up tall with your right foot and right shoulder next to a chair, wall, fence, or other supportive surface for balance.**

2. **Lift your left foot and place your left ankle on the top of your right thigh.**

3. **Inhale and as you exhale, bend your right knee and hinge or bend forward at your hips slightly so your hips move backward, similar to a squat (see Figure 5-7a for an example).**

4. **To deepen the stretch, grab hold of the chair or other supportive surface with both hands (see Figure 5-7b).**

5. **Hold the stretch for 30 seconds or four to five slow, deep breaths.**

6. **Repeat the steps on the other side.**

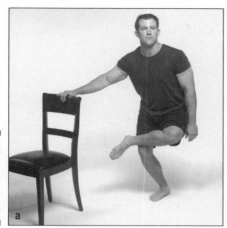 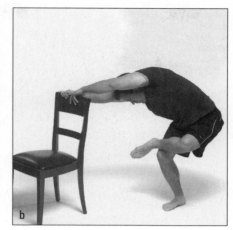

Figure 5-7: Spinal rotation for the back and buttocks.

A few do's and don'ts for this stretch:

- ✔ Do breathe regularly throughout the stretch.
- ✔ Do tilt your pelvis back to feel a deeper stretch in your buttocks.
- ✔ Don't let your knee jut forward; it should stay directly above your ankle. Feel your weight mostly in your heel, not in your toes or the ball of your foot.
- ✔ Don't bounce or force the stretch.

Chapter 6

Soothing Your Lower Back without Paying for a Massage

In This Chapter

▶ Discovering the basic anatomy of the lower back

▶ Focusing on preventing lower back pain

▶ Practicing stretches for a healthy lower back

▶ Releasing tension in your lower back

Accarding to *U.S.News & World Report,* four out of five adults experience significant low back pain at some point in their lives. In addition, back pain is the second most frequent problem that people see their doctor about. For most people under the age of 60, backaches are primarily the result of tight muscles, which create pain that's sudden and short lived — so the good news is that, in most cases, the pain resolves quickly and without intensive therapy or surgery.

However, lower back pain can be a sign of a serious medical condition, so if you have chronic pain in your back, or have currently been experiencing pain in your back for more than three consecutive days, see a doctor before engaging in any of the stretches in this chapter.

In this chapter, I include a routine you can do when you feel general tightness in your lower back, plus I show you some great stretches to do when your back is healthy and you want to keep it that way.

Traveling Around the Lower Back

The five vertebrae that make up the lower back region are called *the lumbar vertebrae,* and they carry the weight of your entire upper body, as well as turn, twist, and bend. Beneath the lumbar vertebrae are nine fused vertebrae that together make up the *sacrum* (the rear wall of the pelvis) and the end of the spine, or the *coccyx.* But these vertebra don't stand up straight all by themselves.

The spine is stabilized primarily by a large muscle group that runs on either side of the spine, known as the erector spinae (shown in Figure 6-1), and by your abdominals. Because no other muscles in your body are capable of such a wide range of movements while supporting such a large weight, they're uniquely susceptible to tension and strain.

The function of all these structures is to maintain good posture (see Figure 6-1). However, as a result of improper movement, muscular imbalance, poor alignment, and/or injury, over time the structures that help maintain fluid movement in your back, such as the intervertebral discs (the soft cartilage between the vertebrae) can begin to be compromised. Because flexibility training can help keep your muscles well balanced and your skeleton properly aligned, stretching is a crucial component of a lifelong commitment to a pain-free and healthy back.

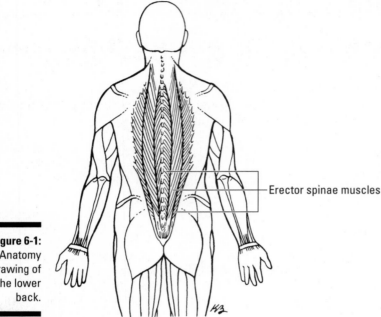

Erector spinae muscles

Figure 6-1:
Anatomy drawing of the lower back.

An Ounce of Prevention Is Worth a Pound of Pain-Free Mobility

I divide the stretches for your lower back into two sections:

- The first includes general stretches to help improve the range of motion and flexibility in your lower back, which can prevent pain and injury to this high-stress area.

- The second section is designed for anyone currently experiencing pain in your lower back. These gentle stretches focus on not only the low back muscles but also surrounding muscles that may be tight and causing low back pain. If you already have the green light from your healthcare professional to try stretching, skip the first section and go directly to the second one.

Seated forward bend

You should feel this stretch along the length of your entire back — specifically the erector spinae. You may hold tension in your upper back and some in your lower back, and because this stretch involves the *entire* back, it can really help you find where you hold tension in your back. For example, if you find that your upper back is tense, that means you hold tension primarily in your rhomboid and trapezious muscles. If your lower back is tense, it's probably your erector spinae that's tight. Either way, this stretch not only helps you increase flexibility in your back, but also it can provide a long-term prescription for back health.

To do this stretch, follow these steps:

1. **Sit on a chair with your feet flat on the floor and your abdominal muscles pulled in.**

   To help you find and control your abdominals, imagine a string attached to your bellybutton. The string pulls back so your bellybutton moves toward your spine. Keep that string tight and your bellybutton pulled in throughout the entire exercise (see Figure 6-2a).

2. **Inhale and as you exhale, bend forward at the hips as far as you can comfortably stretch, letting your arms hang down toward the ground (see Figure 6-2b).**

3. **Hold this stretch for 30 seconds or four to five slow, deep breaths.**

4. **Place your hands on your thighs and slowly roll up one vertebra at a time until you come back to a sitting position.**

To feel a little more stretch in your lats and the middle of your back, after you perform Steps 1 and 2, try to twist your spine slightly so both arms move toward the outside of your right leg. Hold the stretch for 30 seconds and then repeat on your left side.

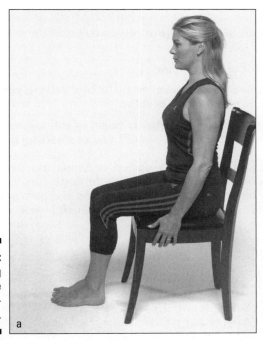 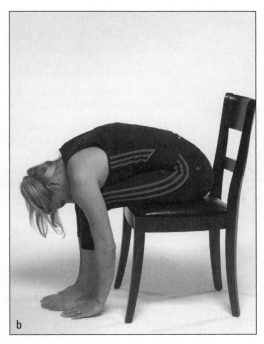

Figure 6-2: Stretching in the seated forward bend.

a   b

A few do's and don'ts for this stretch:

- Do start the motion from your hips, not from your back.
- Do start the stretch in your comfort zone, gradually stretching farther with each breath.
- Don't move or wiggle your legs or knees — your lower body should remain still.
- Don't hold tension in your shoulders.

Standing forward bend

This stretch feels great if your back is tired, especially if you've been standing for a long time. When you stand for an extended period of time, the muscles of your back and hamstrings (the back of your thighs) tend to tighten up, creating stiffness and tension in the muscles. The first phase of this stretch targets the muscles of your back, specifically your erector spinae, and the second phase targets your back and hamstrings.

To do this stretch, follow these steps:

1. **Begin standing with your feet about hip-width apart and your toes facing forward.**

2. **Exhale and bend forward from your hips and knees until your chest rests on your quads and you can place your hands flat on the floor in front of you.**

   Try to keep your hands close to your feet, and your feet flat on the floor (see Figure 6-3a).

3. **Hold this position for 30 seconds.**

   To make sure that the muscles in your neck and shoulders are relaxed, gently shake your head from side to side as if you were saying "no." Remember to breathe as you hold this position.

4. **Exhale and slowly begin straightening your legs until you feel tension in the back of your thighs (see Figure 6-3b).**

   Your hands are still flat on the floor in front of you.

5. **Release the stretch by inhaling, bending your knees again, and resting your torso back on your thighs for the length of two deep breaths.**

6. **Exhale, release your hands from the floor, and slowly begin to roll up, really focusing on stacking your vertebrae — one at a time — until you're standing tall.**

If your back and hamstrings are tight, you may need to place your hands on a yoga block or thick book to keep you from having to bend all the way down to the floor. This assistance allows you to stretch the appropriate muscles without overextending and perhaps causing pain. It's also is a great way to gradually increase your flexibility without overstretching in the beginning.

Figure 6-3:
The standing forward bend — a great lower back and hamstring stretch.

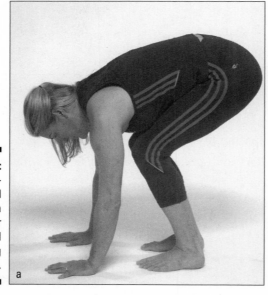
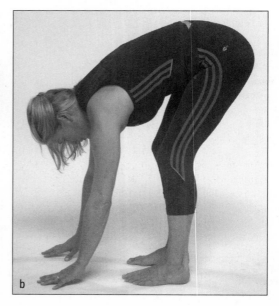

A few do's and don'ts for this stretch:

- ✔ Do keep your hands flat on the floor in front of you and your neck relaxed.
- ✔ Do pull your abdominals in tight when you begin to roll up.
- ✔ Don't tense or tighten your shoulders and/or neck.

Standing pelvic tilts

The standing pelvic tilt helps relieve tightness in your lower back and enhances mobility in the muscles around your pelvis. These muscles include your lower erector spinae, your lower abdominals, and your hip flexors. To see an illustration of where these muscles attach, check out Chapters 5 and 7.

Done properly, the standing pelvic tilt can help improve your sense of body awareness, which results in better posture and less back pain. This stretch requires the use of a wall.

To do this exercise, follow these steps:

1. **Place your back against a wall and walk your feet away from the wall until you can bend your knees so you're in a slight squat.**

   Your back will slide down a few inches as you walk your feet away from the wall. That's okay. Just make sure that you keep your shoulders and hips against the wall the entire time. Notice that there's a slight space between your lower back and the wall. This space is created by the natural curve of your spine.

2. **Rest your hands on your thighs just above your knees.**

3. **Take a deep breath in and as you exhale, slowly tilt your pelvis forward until you feel your lower back against the wall (see Figure 6-4).**

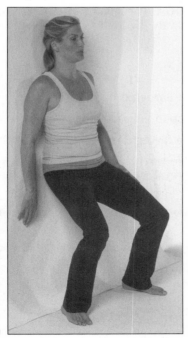

Figure 6-4:
The standing pelvic tilt, using a wall to help you stretch your lower back.

Imagine that you have two flashlights attached to the front of your hipbones. When you tilt your pelvis, the two beams of light should point slightly upward.

4. **Inhale again and release the stretch by moving your pelvis back to the starting position.**

   As the natural curve of your lower back returns, your lower back will move away from the wall.

5. **Exhale and tilt your pelvis again.**

   Repeat the pelvic tilt and release sequence eight to ten times or as many times as feels good to your lower back.

A few do's and don'ts for this exercise:

- ✔ Do hold your abdominals tight. To do so, think of your bellybutton being pulled back toward your spine.

- ✔ Don't try to move your upper body; the movement is in your pelvis.

- ✔ Don't straighten your knees because that decreases the range of motion in your pelvis and makes the stretch less effective. Keep your legs in a slight squat position the entire time.

Shoulder stand with knees bent

If you're looking for an exercise for your back that's a bit more advanced, this stretch is for you. I wouldn't try this stretch if you're a beginner because it requires a bit of strength to be able to hold the position, as well as a good sense of body awareness that only comes with experience. With that said, it's a great stretch for your entire back and neck, focusing especially on lengthening the erector spinae to prevent tightness and injury.

Don't try this stretch if you're new to exercise or stretching. This stretch is advanced and sometimes controversial, so be sure to follow the steps exactly. Avoid rolling too far back so your body weight isn't supported only by your neck. The small vertebrae in your neck weren't made to support the weight of your entire body, so don't risk any strain or injury to your neck.

To do this stretch, follow these steps:

1. **Lie flat on your back on your exercise mat or carpeted floor.**

2. **Bend your knees and pull them all the way up to your chest.**

3. **Rest your arms at your sides with your palms facing down (see Figure 6-5a).**

4. **Inhale and as you exhale, press against the floor with your hands, pull in your abdominals, and lift your hips off the floor so your knees move toward your forehead.**

5. **Lift your hips until your body weight is supported on your shoulder blades (see Figure 6-5b).**

6. **Place your palms against the back of your hips to support the weight of your hips.**

7. **Hold the stretch for 30 seconds, and then slowly roll your body down one vertebra at a time, using your abdominals to control the movement.**

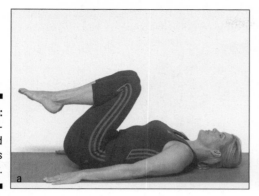 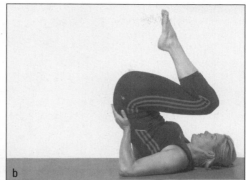

Figure 6-5: The shoulder stand with knees bent.

A few do's and don'ts for this stretch include the following:

🖙 Do support your back with your hands as you hold the stretch.

🖙 Do keep your abdominals tight throughout the entire stretch.

🖙 Do keep your shoulder blades on the floor.

🖙 Don't excessively flex your neck or bring your chin toward your chest.

Opposite arm and leg extension

This stretch help trains all the muscles of your trunk to work together properly to provide stability and balance, while at the same time enhancing flexibility of your erector spinae and abdominals. Remember, keeping your back strong and flexible is the best prevention against low back problems. To do this stretch, follow these steps:

1. **Get on the floor on your hands and knees and lift your abdominals as if your belly-button is lifting toward your spine, while still maintaining neutral spine.**

   Basically, neutral spine is just maintaining the natural curves of your back (not excessively arched or rounded). For more information about neutral spine, see Chapter 2. Make sure to keep your shoulders relaxed, as shown in Figure 6-6a.

2. **At the same time, extend your right arm and your left leg out straight from your body and hold them out about six inches off the floor (see Figure 6-6b).**

   Imagine that strings are attached to your hand and foot and that the strings are gently pulling your arm and leg away from each other, not up. You want to have the sensation of lengthening your spine, not shortening or compressing it.

3. **Hold the stretch for five to eight seconds, breathing comfortably and normally.**

4. **Lower your arm and leg and return to hands and knees on the floor.**

5. **Check to make sure you're still lifting your abdominals, keeping your bellybutton close to your spine and repeat the same exercise with your left arm and right leg.**

6. **Repeat the exercise six or seven more times on each side.**

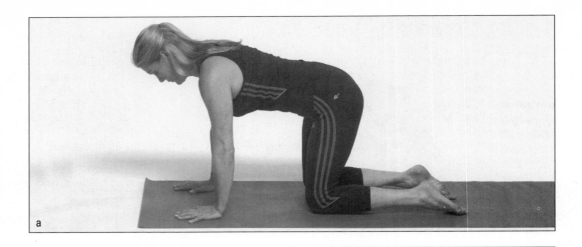

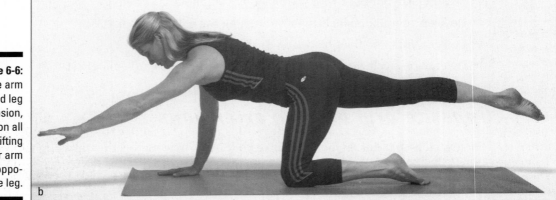

Figure 6-6:
In the arm and leg extension, you're on all fours, lifting your arm and opposite leg.

A few do's and don'ts for this exercise:

✔ Do keep your hips and shoulders level. If your hip of the extended leg is higher than your other hip it may be difficult to keep your balance.

✔ Do keep your abdominals tight. Lax abdominals may place undue stress on your lower back muscles. Your goal is to train your abdominals and back muscles to work together to support your spine.

✔ Don't arch your back.

✔ Don't lift your foot or hand above your hip or shoulder.

Releasing Tension in Your Achy, Breaky Back

The stretches in this section are designed for people who have pain in their lower back as a result of muscle tension. The following five exercises are designed to relieve stress and release muscle tightness in this area.

Alternating knee hugs

This exercise is a rhythmic stretch designed to help you gently stretch your lower back and hamstrings while loosening the hip joint. It's an easy way to slowly get your lower back to release and let go.

To do this exercise, follow these steps:

1. **Lie on your back with your knees bent and your feet flat on the floor.**

2. **Inhale deeply and as you exhale, bring your right knee up toward your c hest, placing your hands behind the knee for guidance and assistance (see Figure 6-7).**

   Don't hold your kneecap — this can cause pressure on and pain in your knee joint.

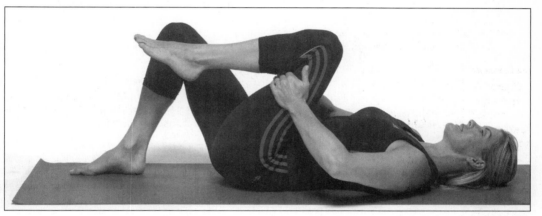

Figure 6-7:
A stretch for your back that involves lying on your back and alternating your knees to your chest.

3. **Hold this stretch for 30 seconds.**

4. **Lower your leg back to the beginning position and repeat the stretch with your left leg.**

5. **Alternate right and left leg stretches for eight to ten repetitions keeping the movement slow and controlled.**

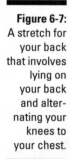

Try this exercise while lying in bed. If your back is so sore that you can't get up and down from the floor, the bed makes a nice substitute for the floor.

A few do's and don'ts for this exercise:

- ✔ Do exhale as you bring your knee forward.
- ✔ Do keep your neck and shoulders relaxed.
- ✔ Don't bring your knee so far toward your chest that the movement causes your hips to lift off the floor.

The tennis ball massage

Sometimes muscles that have been very tight for a long period of time can actually lose the ability to relax on their own, resulting in persistent muscle and skeletal imbalance, nerve impingement, and most likely, chronic pain. When that happens, the only thing that can really help the muscle let go is focused massage. Unfortunately, for most people a good massage is a luxury of both time and money. But don't despair — one of the most effective methods I've found to apply pinpoint massage on chronically tight and painful muscles is both quick and inexpensive. All you need is a tennis ball and an open space on the floor.

Two techniques are useful and both are simple. Here's the first one:

1. Place a tennis ball on a clean, flat place on the floor, and lie down with the ball directly beneath your tight muscle.

2. Lie there and breathe deeply, using your own body weight to apply pressure to the muscle while the increased amount of oxygen in your blood helps to initiate the relaxation response and to wash through the tight muscle and remove toxins.

The second goes like this:

1. Place a tennis ball on a clean, flat place on the floor, and lie down with the ball directly beneath your tight muscle.

2. Move slowly back and forth, gently rolling the tennis ball all around the affected area to mimic the motion of a firm, steady massage.

   Do this for approximately 30 seconds, and then roll off the tight area to give it a rest.

3. Repeat until you feel the muscle relax.

I do want to give you two precautions with this massage technique:

✔ Don't overdo it. Let the muscle relax slowly and gradually. It may take repeated attempts over several days to get severely tight muscles to stop clenching and let go. Aggressive massage can actually bruise the muscle, which just makes things worse and keeps you from addressing your fundamental muscle tension for several days until you heal.

✔ Never place the ball directly beneath your spine. Your spine is made of bones, and bones won't stretch. They can bruise, though, and be pushed out of alignment, which again will only make things worse.

As a program of preventive treatment, keep a tennis ball handy, and stretch out on the floor whenever you feel tightness building up. These measures will keep you out of the doctor's office and make your next massage all about indulgence, not pain management.

Mini back massage

This stretch is my all-time favorite stretch for my lower back. Because your back is against the floor during this exercise, your back muscles don't have to work to hold you upright and can now completely relax and let go.

To do this exercise, follow these steps:

1. **Lie flat on your back and bring both knees toward your chest, placing your hands under each knee for support (see Figure 6-8a).**

2. **Breathe deeply and slowly rock side to side, feeling the floor against the right and left side of your lower back.**

   This movement should give your lower back a gentle massage. Hug your knees for an extra stretch as you rock side to side (see Figure 6-8b).

3. **As you rock, hold the stretch for 30 to 60 seconds, depending on your level of comfort.**

If for any reason it's uncomfortable to get to the floor, you can still do this stretch in bed. You won't feel the massage as strongly, but you will still get a nice gentle stretch for your sore back.

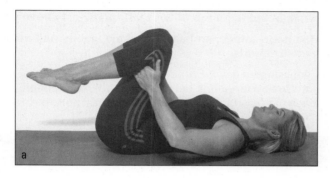

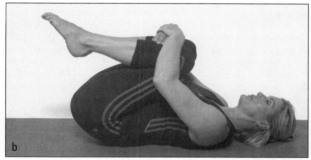

Figure 6-8: The mini back massage uses the floor to gently massage your back.

A few do's and don'ts for this exercise:

- Do breath slowly and rhythmically.

- Do grasp your knees with both hands and pull them into your chest for a deeper stretch.

- Don't rock your hips so far to each side that you loose your balance. Your knees should only move a few inches in each direction and your hips should never leave the floor.

Lying buttocks and hip stretch, legs crossed

I've included this stretch for your buttocks because oftentimes low back pain can actually be caused by a tight muscle that affects the low back area. Tight muscles that affect your back include calves, hamstrings, buttocks, and hip flexors. If these muscles are tight they can pull on surrounding muscles, causing your lower back to overcompensate, creating poor posture and muscular imbalance.

This specific stretch targets your piriformis, which is a muscle in your buttocks that when tight can pinch your sciatic nerve, causing pain. Because all your muscles attach to each other and affect each other, maintaining flexibility in all the areas surrounding your lower back can go a long way toward fighting low back pain.

To do this stretch, follow these steps:

1. **Lie on your back with your knees bent and feet flat on the floor.**

   You can perform this stretch lying in bed if it is more comfortable for you.

2. **Place the outside of your right ankle on top of your left thigh, just above your knee.**

3. **Raise your left foot off the floor, inhale, and as you exhale, gently pull your left knee closer to your chest with your hands.**

   Don't forget to interlock your fingers *behind* your left knee for support (see Figure 6-9a). If it's uncomfortable to interlock your hands behind your knee, try wrapping a small hand towel around the back of your thigh and use that to gently pull your leg toward your chest.

4. **With your right elbow, gently press your right knee away from you (see Figure 6-9b).**

5. **Hold the stretch for 30 seconds, gradually deepening the stretch with every exhalation.**

6. **Repeat the stretch by switching legs.**

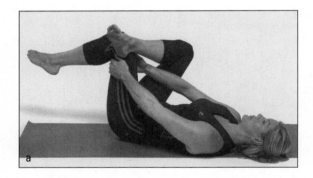

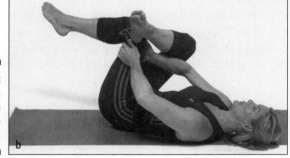

Figure 6-9:
The lying
buttocks
and hip
stretch.

A few do's and don'ts for this stretch:

✔ Do keep your shoulder blades down and your upper body relaxed.

✔ Do be patient and let the stretch deepen with each breath.

✔ Don't lift your hips off the floor or lean to one side.

✔ Don't bounce or force the stretch.

The cow and the cat

This yoga-based move got its name from imagining what an old cow and an angry cat look like. Not only does this move help make your back feel better, but also it improves the range of motion in your spine, enhances strength and coordination of the muscles around your spine, and improves muscle awareness in your entire back — all factors that make your lower back feel better and stay healthy.

To do this stretch, follow these steps:

1. **Get on the floor on your hands and knees with your hands directly under your shoulders and your knees directly under your hips.**

2. **Lay the tops of your feet on the floor and point your toes back.**

3. **Inhale and arch your back, lifting your tailbone and eyes toward the ceiling (see Figure 6-10a).**

4. **Hold the stretch for a few seconds, release the position back to neutral spine, and then inhale again.**

5. **Exhale and contract your abdominals, rounding your back like an angry cat (see Figure 6-10b).**

6. **Hold this position for a few seconds and then release back to neutral spine.**

7. **Repeat this stretch four to six times.**

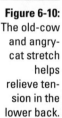

Figure 6-10: The old-cow and angry-cat stretch helps relieve tension in the lower back.

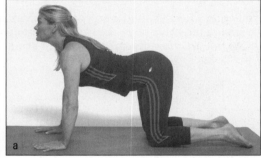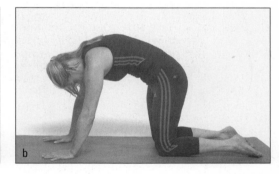

A few do's and don'ts for this exercise:

- ✓ Do pull your bellybutton toward your spine.

- ✓ Do keep the movement in your pelvis and lower back, not in your shoulders.

- ✓ Don't tense up your shoulders and neck.

- ✓ Don't overextend your neck while doing the old cow position.

Hip flexor stretch on one knee

Because your hip flexor muscles run across the front of your hip and attach to your lower back, tight hip flexor muscles may be a hidden source of lower back tension. This stretch helps lengthen the iliopsoas (il-ee-oh-*so*-as) and relaxes your lower back.

A little TLC for your back

According to the American Academy of Orthopedic Surgeons (AAOS), four out of five adults experience significant low back pain sometime during their life. Work-related back injuries are the nation's number-one occupational hazard, but you can suffer back pain from activities at home and at play, too. The AAOS has developed the following tips to help reduce the risk of back pain when lifting and moving any kind of heavy weight:

✔ When standing, spread your feet shoulder-width apart to give yourself a solid base of support and then slightly bend your knees.

✔ Tighten your stomach muscles before lifting.

✔ Position the person or object close to your body before lifting.

✔ Lift with your leg muscles. Never lift an object by keeping your legs stiff, while bending over it.

✔ Avoid twisting your body; instead, point your toes in the direction you want to move and pivot in that direction.

✔ When placing an object on a high shelf, move close to the shelf.

✔ During lifting movements, maintain the natural curve of your spine; don't bend at your waist.

✔ Do not try to lift something that is too heavy by yourself or that is an awkward shape. Get help.

For more information, check out the AAOS Web site at www.aaos.org.

To do this stretch, follow these steps:

1. **Kneel on your left knee.**

2. **Bend your right knee, and place your right foot flat on the floor (see Figure 6-11).**

   Make sure your abdominals are pulled in, chest is lifted, and your shoulder blades are down. Check to see if your shoulders are directly above your hips. Maintaining good posture with your upper body allows you to correctly stretch without straining.

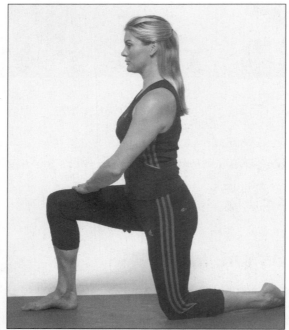

Figure 6-11: The kneeling hip flexor stretch.

3. **Inhale and as you exhale, squeeze your buttocks and tilt your pelvis forward so that the front of your hipbones tilt slightly upward.**

   You should feel this stretch in the front part of your right hip.

4. **Hold this stretch for 30 seconds or four to five slow, deep breaths.**

5. **Repeat Steps 1 through 3, bending the left leg and kneeling on the right knee.**

   If this stretch is uncomfortable on the knee supporting your weight, try placing a folded towel or pillow under your knee as a cushion.

A few do's and don'ts for this stretch:

- ✔ Do breathe rhythmically and deeply throughout the stretch.
- ✔ Do keep your shoulders directly over your hips so the front of your hip is lengthened, not shortened.
- ✔ Do focus on squeezing your buttocks and tilting your pelvis forward.
- ✔ Don't hinge forward at your hips.
- ✔ Don't arch your back.

Chapter 7

From Your Knickers to Your Kickers: Stretches for your Bottom Half

- -

In This Chapter

▶ Getting familiar with the muscles of your lower body

▶ Loosening up your hips and buttocks

▶ Stretching your thighs

▶ Performing lower leg stretches

▶ Taking care of your feet and ankles

- -

The muscles of your lower body — your hips, buttocks, thighs, calves, ankles, and feet — all work together like the many different instruments in an orchestra. When they're all doing their part, they make beautiful music together, but when one of them is out of tune, the entire performance suffers.

Tightness in the lower body can be the hidden culprit in a wide variety of ailments that, at first glance, you may not blame them for. Poor posture, disorders of the back such as lordosis (swayback) or scoliosis (lateral curvature of the spine), indigestion, headaches, and even difficulty breathing can all be caused to one degree or another by imbalances in the lower body due to muscle tension and tightness.

For yet another example, a runner with tight hamstrings can have a shortened stride due to the tightness. A shortened stride means more steps, which means expending more energy, which means energy wasted. It also means more impact, which can lead to more injuries. But stretching can stop this cycle of doom, once and for all.

In this chapter, I break down the muscles of the lower body into sections: hips and buttocks, hamstrings, quadriceps, groin and inner thigh, lower leg, and feet and ankles. Each section gives you a variety of stretches for that particular area. Experiment with each stretch to see which stretches suit your body best.

Throughout the following stretches for your hips, buttocks, and thighs, be aware of the position of your pelvis (see Figure 7-1). All these muscles are attached to your pelvis in one way or another, and if your pelvis isn't correctly positioned, you can diminish the effectiveness of these stretches. To improve your body awareness in this area, try doing the pelvic tilts I describe in Chapter 8.

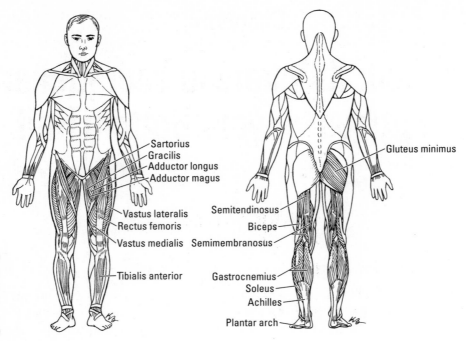

Figure 7-1:
The muscles of your lower half.

Sartorius
Gracilis
Adductor longus
Adductor magus

Vastus lateralis
Rectus femoris

Vastus medialis

Tibialis anterior

Gluteus minimus

Semitendinosus

Biceps

Semimembranosus

Gastrocnemius
Soleus
Achilles

Plantar arch

Behind the Scenes: Hips and Buttocks

What does an athlete who never stretches and a dedicated couch potato have in common? If you said they both really need to read this book, you're right! But another answer is that even though one is actually an athlete, they both probably have tight hip flexors.

To enhance your wealth of knowledge about your body, here are a few terms to tuck away regarding the hip and buttocks muscles and their functional roles (no, not the role of swaying to and fro to attract that special someone's attention):

✔ **Hip flexors:** These muscles are also known as the iliopsoas (il-ee-oh-*so*-as) and are made up of three muscles — the psoas (*so*-as) major, psoas minor, and iliacus (*il*-ee-ah-kus) that run across the front of the hip and pass through the pelvis, attaching to your lower back area. They work together to flex the hips and rotate the lower spine.

This area can get very tight because it gets a lot of use. The hip flexors are the muscles that lift your knee or move your leg forward is such movements as going up stairs, walking, running, or just about anything that has to do with forward motion. Ironically, these muscles can also get tight and shorten if you sit all day. And, because this muscle group attaches to your lower back area, if it is tight it can cause lower back pain.

✔ **Glutes:** One of the primary muscles of the buttocks; "glutes" is slang that collectively refers to the three muscles in the buttocks:

• **Gluteus maximus:** The largest and most superficial muscle in your buttocks, the maximus is responsible for hip extension, and it also helps rotate the hip outward.

• **Gluteus medius:** This muscle is the mid-size glute, and its function is to move your leg to the side (abduction of your hip joint). It also helps rotate your thigh inward and outward.

• **Gluteus minimus:** The smallest and deepest of the glutes. It also functions as a hip abductor and rotates the thigh inward and outward.

✔ **Piriformis:** The piriformis (peer-i-*for*-mus) plays an important role in stabilizing the spine, working together with the iliopsoas to create pelvic balance.

If either the iliopsoas or the piriformis is excessively tight or weak, you can experience low back pain or other postural problems. That's why it's important to balance the strength and flexibility of the iliopsoas muscle (front of the hip) with the strength and flexibility of the glutes and piriformis (buttocks).

The following stretches give you several options to stretch the entire hip and buttocks area.

Runner's lunge

The runner's lunge is one of the best stretches for everyone, not just runners. The stretch targets your iliopsoas. Because of the importance of these muscles to your back health and overall leg health, no matter what, stretching this area is a must.

If this stretch is uncomfortable for you to get into, try doing it with your back leg extended on an exercise bench and your front foot on the floor.

To do this stretch, follow these steps:

1. **Begin standing with your legs spread about two feet apart with the right foot in front of you and the left foot behind you (see Figure 7-2a).**

2. **Inhale and as you exhale, bend both knees until you can place both hands on the floor directly behind your right heel.**

3. **Slide your left leg back far enough so you can lower your knee to the floor without putting weight on your kneecap (see Figure 7-2b).**

4. **Inhale again and as you exhale gently press the front of the hip of your left leg toward the floor.**

5. **Hold this stretch for 30 seconds or four to five slow, deep breaths.**

6. **Repeat the same stretch on the right side.**

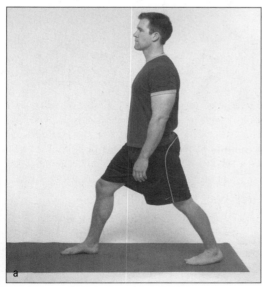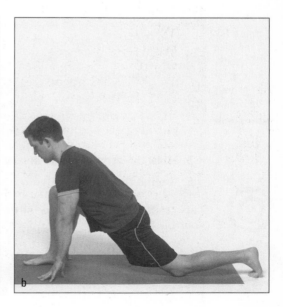

Figure 7-2: Stretching your iliopsoas in the runner's lunge.

A few do's and don'ts for this stretch:

- ✔ Do keep your chest lifted and your shoulder blades down.
- ✔ Do keep your front knee at a right angle and directly over your front heel.
- ✔ Do progress through the stretch gradually and slowly.
- ✔ Don't jut your front knee forward — if your front knee is moving forward, you could be putting undue strain on your knee.
- ✔ Don't put your weight on the kneecap of the leg behind you. Instead, your weight should be supported on the softer part of your leg just above your kneecap.

Lying buttocks stretch with foot to opposite shoulder

This lying buttocks stretch specifically targets your gluteus maximus. To do this stretch, follow these steps:

1. **Lie on your back with your legs straight out in front of you.**
2. **Bring your right knee toward your chest, keeping your left leg straight.**
3. **With your right hand, hold your knee (on top of the knee) and grab your right ankle with your left hand.**
4. **Inhale and as you exhale pull your foot toward your opposite shoulder and your knee toward the midline of your body (see Figure 7-3).**

   Make sure to keep your shoulders and head on the floor.

Figure 7-3: The lying buttocks stretch for your gluteus maximus.

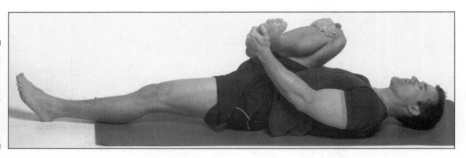

5. **Hold the stretch for 30 seconds or four to five deep breaths.**
6. **Repeat the stretch on your left side.**

This stretch can also be done sitting with your back against a wall, but remember to keep your back upright and your opposite leg straight.

A few do's and don'ts for this stretch:

- ✔ Do keep your shoulders and head on the floor.
- ✔ Do breathe throughout the stretch.

✔ Do progress through the stretch gradually and slowly.

✔ Don't pull on your foot only; this places undue stress on your knee.

✔ Don't tuck your pelvis under — think of tilting your tailbone toward the floor.

Buttocks stretch

Believe it or not, nine muscles make up the buttocks area. And, believe it or not, this lying hip and buttocks stretch lengthens them *all* — even the smaller, deeper muscles.

If your buttocks is tight, specifically your piriformis muscle, it can pinch your sciatic nerve and cause pain similar to sciatica. This stretch specifically targets the piriformis.

To do this stretch, follow these steps:

1. **Lie on your back with your knees bent and feet flat on the floor.**

2. **Lift your right foot and place the outside of your right ankle on your left thigh, just above your knee.**

3. **Raise your left foot off the floor, inhale, and as you exhale, gently pull your left knee closer to your chest with your hands (see Figure 7-4a).**

   Don't forget to interlock your fingers *behind* your left knee for support. If it's uncomfortable to interlock your hands behind your knee, try wrapping a small hand towel around the back of your thigh and use that to gently pull your leg toward your chest.

4. **With your right elbow, gently press your right knee away from you (see Figure 7-4b).**

5. **Hold the stretch for 30 seconds, gradually deepening the stretch with every exhalation.**

6. **Repeat the stretch by switching legs.**

Figure 7-4:
The lying buttocks and hip stretch with your legs crossed.

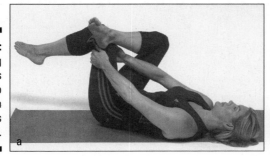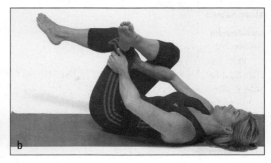

A few do's and don'ts for this stretch:

✔ Do keep your shoulder blades down and your upper body relaxed.

✔ Do be patient and let the stretch deepen with each breath.

✔ Don't lift your hips off the floor or lean to one side.

✔ Don't bounce or force the stretch.

Seated external rotator stretch

Dancers love this stretch because it targets the muscles that outwardly rotate the hips and thighs — your gluteus medius and gluteus minimus (muscles that get used a lot if you're a *ballet* dancer). As an added bonus, you get a nice stretch in your core muscles, too.

To do this stretch, follow these steps:

1. **Sit on the floor with your right leg straight in front of you and your left foot crossed over your right thigh.**

2. **As you inhale, pull your left knee toward your chest with your right hand and sit up very straight as if a string was attached to the top of your head, lengthening your spine (see Figure 7-5a).**

3. **As you exhale, look over your left shoulder, rotating your spine and tilting your pelvis back (see Figure 7-5b).**

4. **Hold the stretch for about 30 seconds, deepening the stretch with every breath.**

   Feel this stretch in your buttocks and pay close attention to the position of your pelvis. Imagine a string attached to your tailbone pulling your tailbone toward the back wall.

5. **Switch sides and repeat the same stretch on your other leg.**

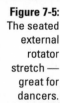

Figure 7-5:
The seated external rotator stretch — great for dancers.

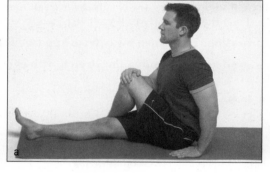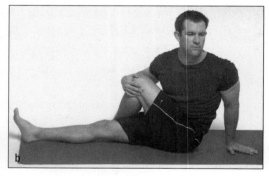

A few do's and don'ts for this stretch:

- ✔ Do bring your knee close to your chest *before* you twist.
- ✔ Do look over your shoulder so you lengthen your neck muscles as well.
- ✔ Do sit up straight to lengthen your spine *before* you rotate.
- ✔ Don't tuck your pelvis under or round your back.

Tight End: Back of the Thigh

Three primary muscles bend your knee and extend your hip: the biceps femoris (*fem*-er-is), the semitendinosus (semi-ten-duh-*no*-sis), and the semimembranosus (semi-mem-bruh-*no*-sis). Together, these three muscles are collectively known as your hamstrings. All of them are found next to each other in the back of your thigh.

Because you use your hamstrings for just about every movement your legs make, an injury to this area takes a long time to heal, and these muscles are easy to reinjure. A pulled hamstring can sideline you for a long time — just ask any professional athlete what a "pain in the butt" it is! So it's important to do all you can to avoid a strain or pull in this area.

A hamstring pull — a strain injury caused by a violent overextension or rapid contraction of the muscle — could be caused by an imbalance of strength between your hamstrings and your quadriceps or because of an imbalance of strength between your right and left leg. But in most cases the cause of the injury is a fundamental lack of flexibility. Keeping your hamstrings flexible is your best defense against this type of injury. So get stretching!

Lying leg extension

The lying leg extension is one of the easiest positions in which to isolate your hamstrings without having any other muscles pulling or straining. If you know you have tight hamstrings, I recommend using a towel or stretching strap (as I mention in Chapter 2) to help keep your upper body relaxed and tension free.

If your hamstrings are extremely tight, you may find it more comfortable to do this stretch lying in a doorway with one leg on the floor and the other leg extended and resting against the doorjamb. As you get more flexible, your hips will get closer to the wall.

To do this stretch, follow these steps:

1. **Lie on your back with your feet flat on the floor and close to your buttocks.**

2. **Lift your right leg and extend it upward (see Figure 7-6a).**

3. **Place one hand behind your thigh and one hand behind your knee or calf.**

   Try to keep your leg straight but remember to stay in your comfort zone.

4. **Inhale and as you exhale gently pull your leg closer toward your shoulders (see Figure 7-6b).**

   Remember to keep your shoulders on the ground. Feel the stretch deepen with every exhale until you've reached the deepest point of the stretch.

5. **Hold the stretch for 30 seconds or four to five slow, deep breaths.**

6. **Repeat the stretch on your other leg.**

Figure 7-6:
The lying leg extension.

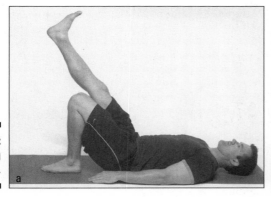
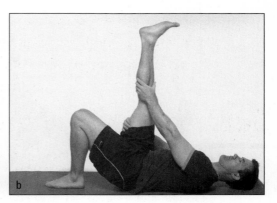

Your goal is to feel the stretch in the back of your thigh, not to get your knee to your nose. It's important to anchor your hips to the floor, not to tuck your pelvis under or round your back. Don't worry about how far down your leg gets; just feel the stretch in your hamstring.

A few do's and don'ts for this stretch:

- ✔ Do breathe as you hold the stretch.
- ✔ Do progress through the stretch gradually.
- ✔ Do lie comfortably on the floor with your arms and shoulders relaxed.
- ✔ Don't tuck your hips under or lift them off the floor.
- ✔ Don't bend your knee.

Standing stretch with foot on chair

If getting on the ground is uncomfortable or inconvenient for you, try out this hamstring stretch. You can use a chair or bench or even a fence if you've just finished running outdoors. Just make sure that where you place your foot is no higher than your hips.

To do this stretch, follow these steps:

1. **Stand up straight with your feet flat on the floor and your abdominals lifted.**

2. **Lift your right leg and rest it on a chair or bench straight in front of you.**

   Keep your hips squared to the front and both legs straight (see Figure 7-7a).

3. **Inhale and as you exhale, lean forward from your hips and feel the stretch deepen in the back of your thigh (see Figure 7-7b).**

   Avoid rounding or bending your back.

4. **Hold the stretch for 30 seconds or four to five slow, deep breaths.**

5. **Repeat this stretch on the other leg.**

Figure 7-7: Stretching your hamstrings in a more comfortable position.

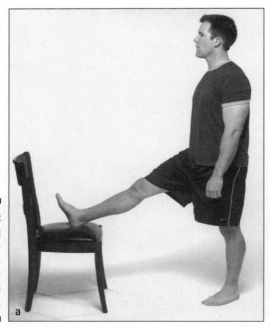
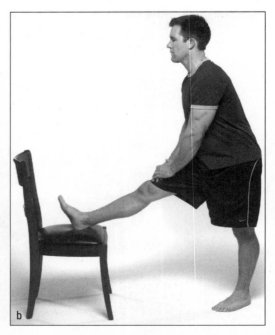

One trick I use to get a muscle group to relax is to contract the opposing muscle group. Try contracting your quadriceps (the muscles in the front of your thigh) while you stretch your hamstrings (the back of your thigh). This can help relax your hamstrings while you hold this stretch, and if your hamstrings are relaxed you get a deeper stretch.

A few do's and don'ts for this stretch:

✔ Do breathe as you hold the stretch.

✔ Do progress through the stretch gradually.

✔ Do tilt your pelvis back, not under.

✔ Don't round or bend at your waist; hinge at the hips and keep your back straight.

Modified hurdler stretch

You may remember the hurdler stretch from PE class, sitting on the grass with your bent knee twisted behind you. Fitness folks now know that that extreme position can put a lot of stress on your knee. I hope you find this modification more comfortable and less risky. You also get the added benefit of stretching your back and calf muscles, too.

This stretch is more comfortable and effective to perform by using the aid of a towel or stretching strap (see Chapter 2 for more details on straps).

To do this stretch, follow these steps:

1. **Sit on the floor with your right leg straight out in front of you, your left leg bent inward at a comfortable angle, and your arms to your sides (see Figure 7-8a).**

2. **As you exhale, hinge forward at the hip, keeping your right leg straight and your foot relaxed.**

3. **Reach forward toward your toes as far as you can without bending your knee.**

   If your right knee begins to bend or your upper back begins to tighten and get tense, you have gone too far. See Figure 7-8b for a visual of this stretching motion. You can also imagine your tailbone moving toward the back of the room and your heel reaching toward the front of the room. This visualization should help you lengthen the back of your leg from both directions. Your tailbone should be reaching back as you hinge forward at the hips.

4. **Breathe deeply and hold the stretch for 30 seconds.**

   Deepen the stretch with each breath by tilting your pelvis back, lifting your chest, and flexing your foot so your toes are moving toward your shoulders.

5. **Switch sides and repeat the same stretch on your other leg.**

Figure 7-8:
The modified hurdler stretch that doesn't hurt your knees.

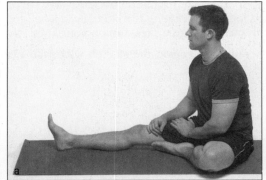
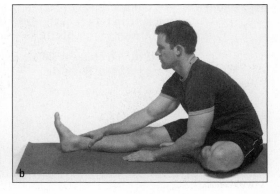

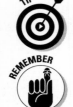

If you have trouble keeping your shoulders and neck relaxed, try hooking a towel or stretching strap (described in Chapter 2) around the ball of your foot and then gently pulling on the ends of the towel/strap. Don't get discouraged if your chest is nowhere near your leg. As long as you're feeling a good deep stretch in the back of your thigh, you're doing great!

A few do's and don'ts for this stretch:

- ✔ Do gently hinge forward at your hips with your eyes looking forward.
- ✔ Do keep your knee straight, and try to keep the back of your knee on the floor.
- ✔ Do keep your back straight, not rounded, and don't tense your shoulders.
- ✔ Don't bounce or force the stretch.
- ✔ Don't look down at your knee; look at the floor in front of your toes.

Forward Thinking: Front of Thighs

The front of your thigh is a group of four muscles that work together known as the quadriceps (called *quads* for short): the rectus femoris, vastus lateralis, vastus medialis, and the vastus intermedius. Their main function is to extend your knee, so that means that they get used a lot. If these muscles get excessively tight, they can pull unevenly on your knee joint, which can cause knee pain. The stretches in this section show you how to stretch and lengthen your quads.

Ankle to buttocks, on your side

Give yourself a kick in the buttocks (literally) with this quad stretch. Okay, it's really not that hard. This stretch has you lying on your side, and contains two unique features: It's one of the most accessible quad stretches to get into, and after you're in it, proper form is easy to maintain. I recommend this stretch if you're new to stretching.

To do this stretch, follow these steps:

1. **Start by lying on your right side with your knees bent close to your chest.**

2. **Rest your right arm comfortably in a bent position underneath your head (to support your head) — see Figure 7-9a.**

3. **Grab the top of your left foot and gently pull your ankle back toward your buttocks (see Figure 7-9b).**

   You should feel the stretch in the front of your thigh. If you squeeze your buttocks, you can increase the stretch, but don't let your hips roll back. Always keep your hips stacked on top of each other, and focus on bringing the knee back. Don't force your heel toward your buttocks, which can put undue pressure on your knee joint.

4. **Hold the stretch for 30 seconds, and then repeat the stretch with your right leg and lying on your left side.**

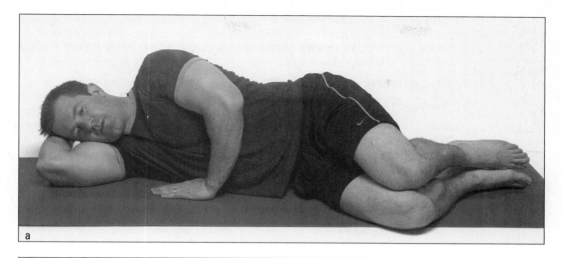

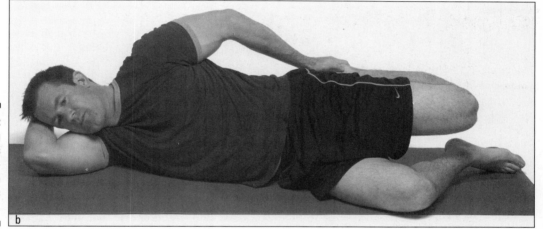

Figure 7-9:
Stretching
your quads
in a side-
lying ankle
to buttocks
stretch.

A few do's and don'ts for this stretch:

- Do breathe as you hold the stretch.
- Do squeeze your buttocks and slightly tuck your pelvis under to deepen the stretch.
- Do keep your bottom knee bent for balance.
- Don't jam your heel toward your buttocks.
- Don't hold your breath.
- Don't lift the knee — try to keep your inner thighs touching each other.

Heel to buttocks, facedown

If your quads are stiff or sore *after* a workout, try this stretch as a cool-down to further stretch and relax your muscles.

To do this stretch, follow these steps:

1. **Lie on the floor, facedown with both legs straight out behind your body and your left hand at your side.**

2. **Make a fist with your right hand and rest your forehead on your fist.**

3. **Bend your left knee and raise your heel toward your buttocks.**

4. **Reach back with your left hand and grab the top of your left foot and hold the foot in place (see Figure 7-10).**

   If you have difficulty reaching the top of your foot, grab the back of your heel, ankle, or even the hem of your pant leg. But don't pull down on your foot. Instead, just rest your foot in your hand as you focus on pressing your hip to the floor. This should keep the stretch in your quads, not in your knee joint.

Figure 7-10: A good stretch for your quads.

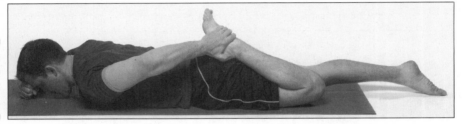

5. **Inhale and as you exhale squeeze your buttocks and gently press your hip toward the floor.**

   Avoid letting your left knee move out to the side as you reach for it with your left hand. Try to keep your knees as close together as you can; this position avoids misalignment, which can cause stress to your knee joint.

6. **Hold the stretch for 30 seconds or four to five slow, deep breaths.**

7. **Repeat Steps 1 through 6 with your right leg.**

A few do's and don'ts for this stretch:

- ✔ Do keep your head down and resting on your fist.
- ✔ Do breathe to relax into the stretch.
- ✔ Do keep your knees together and squeeze your buttocks.
- ✔ Do focus on pressing your hip toward the floor.
- ✔ Don't focus on bringing your foot to your buttocks.

Standing stretch, knee toward buttocks

This stretch is a great standing stretch that targets your quads. Because this stretch is done standing, it's probably the most practical and convenient stretch to do *after* you've been exercising outdoors because you won't need to lie down on the wet grass or muddy ground. To do this stretch, follow these steps:

1. **Stand up tall and place your right hand on a stable surface.**

   The surface can be a chair, wall, doorway, or fence — anything that's sturdy and helps you keep your balance during this stretch.

2. **Inhale and lift your left knee toward the sky and grab hold of your left ankle (or top of your foot) with your left hand (see Figure 7-11a).**

3. **Exhale and slowly lower your left knee and gently move your left foot toward your left buttocks (see Figure 7-11b).**

   Try to keep the inside of your thighs touching and focus on moving your knee back, not forcing your foot to touch your buttocks. To really feel this stretch correctly, try to tuck your pelvis under and think about your tailbone moving toward the floor.

4. **Hold this stretch for 30 seconds or about four to five slow, deep breaths.**

5. **Repeat the stretch with the right leg.**

To make this exercise one for balance as well, try to let go of the stable surface and see if you can hold your balance as you continue to stretch your quadriceps.

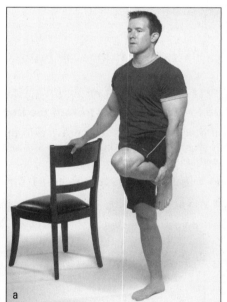 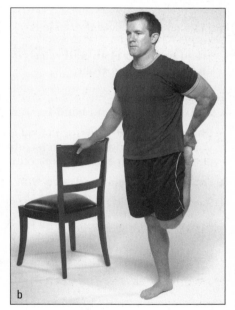

Figure 7-11: The standing quad stretch.

a   b

A few do's and don'ts for this stretch:

✔ Do stand up tall with your chest lifted, abs in, and shoulder blades down to help you feel the stretch correctly and practice good posture, too!

✔ Do tilt your pelvis under.

✔ Don't put undue stress on your knee by forcing your foot to touch your buttocks.

✔ Don't let your knee move to the side; keep the insides of your legs touching.

Becoming Master of Your Inner Thighs

Five muscles make up the area commonly known as the groin. These muscles are the adductor longus, adductor brevis, adductor magnus, gracilis, and pectineus. To simplify things, just call them your adductors or inner thigh muscles. Like your hamstrings, these muscles are involved in almost every movement of your legs, and if they're tight, they may be prone to injuries, which are awkward to treat. Your best bet to avoid this difficult and painful situation is not only to keep these muscles strong but also to stretch them regularly.

Standing groin stretch

Your adductors are the muscles that run along your inner thighs and groin. Although there are many different ways to stretch your adductors, this stretch is probably the easiest way to stretch your entire groin area without tensing your neck, shoulders, and back.

Grab a chair for this exercise — and make sure that the chair is sturdy and stable. No rolling office chairs for this stretch!

To do this stretch, follow these steps:

1. **Stand next to a chair and raise your leg that's closest to the chair to place your foot on the seat of the chair.**

   Make sure to keep your hips and shoulders facing forward, as shown in Figure 7-12a.

2. **Exhale slowly as you bend forward and lower your hands toward the floor.**

   Check out Figure 7-12b for the visualization of this stretch. Let gravity do the work — you shouldn't have to. If you feel too much strain, place one hand on the seat of the chair to give you a little more control over the stretch.

3. **Gradually deepen the stretch with every exhale as you hold this stretch for 30 seconds.**

   Shake your head "no" to make sure that you aren't holding tension in your neck.

4. **Roll up slowly and repeat the stretch with your other leg.**

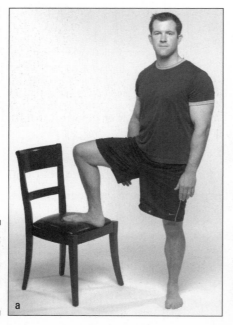
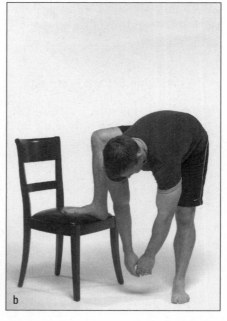

Figure 7-12: Standing forward bend with chair.

a

b

A few do's and don'ts for this stretch:

✔ Do tilt your pelvis back so you feel the stretch a little deeper in your groin.

✔ Don't rush!

✔ Don't bounce or force the stretch because those motions can cause the muscles to tighten up rather than relax and lengthen.

Seated straddle stretch

Even though this is a common stretch, because of the complexity of all the muscles involved it's not an easy stretch to do properly. Your hamstrings, back, and inner thighs must all work together to perform this stretch with good form. If any of these areas are tight the effectiveness of the stretch can be compromised.

To do this stretch, follow these steps:

1. **Sit on the floor with your legs straight and your feet as far apart as possible.**

2. **Place your hands behind your hips and sit up very tall.**

   Keeping your hands behind your hips helps you keep your spine lifted and straight, allowing you to stretch your back, inner thighs, and hamstrings without creating tension in your shoulders and upper back.

3. **Move your hips forward an inch or two until you feel the stretch along both inner thighs (see Figure 7-13a).**

4. **Inhale, and as you exhale, lean slightly forward, tilting your pelvis back (see Figure 7-13b).**

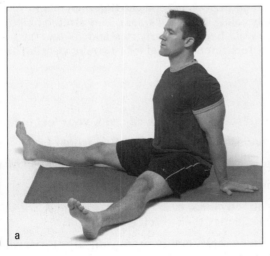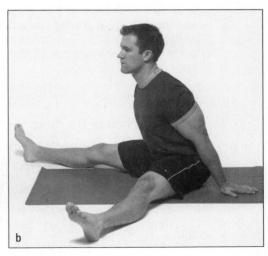

Figure 7-13: The seated straddle stretch.

a

b

5. **Hold the stretch for 30 seconds or four to five slow, deep breaths.**

If keeping your back straight and your hips tilted back is difficult, try performing this stretch while sitting on a pillow or folded towel or blanket. By raising your hips off the floor, some stress on your hamstrings will ease, allowing you to focus on your inner thighs.

A few do's and don'ts for this stretch:

- Do keep your knees and toes facing upward toward the ceiling.
- Do tilt your pelvis back as you lift your chest.
- Do breathe deeply through the entire stretch.
- Don't place your hands in front of you unless you can keep them there without rounding your spine or tucking your pelvis under.
- Don't bounce this stretch.

Putting Your Best Foot (And Lower Leg) Forward

Your lower leg is basically made up of the area between your knee and ankle — specifically your calf and shin. Many little muscles make up your calf, but the two muscles I think you should be aware of are your *gastrocnemius* (gas-trok-*nee*-mee-uhs) and your *soleus* (*soh*-lee-uhs). The gastrocnemius pretty much defines your calf and the soleus is the smaller muscle under your gastrocnemius). These two muscles do most of the work of pointing your foot downward, including pushing off when you walk, run, or jump. Because these muscles attach to your heel with your Achilles tendon, if these muscles are excessively tight, they can put undue stress on your Achilles tendon, and you know what happened to Achilles!

Standing calf stretch

Wearing high heels and standing for long periods of time can tighten and shorten your calf muscles, which over time can actually cause lower back pain. This stretch helps keep you limber if you're one of the many who wear heels regularly or stand all day. Try to find a moment several times during the day to stretch your calves (if you're wearing heels, take them off first!).

To do this exercise, follow these steps:

1. **Face a wall or sturdy surface and stand one foot away with your feet together.**

2. **Lean forward and place your hands directly on the wall in front of you.**

3. **Move your left foot back as far as you can while still keeping your heel on the floor.**

4. **Bend the right knee slightly but keep the left knee straight.**

   Try to keep your toes pointing directly forward in line with your heel. The more you turn your toes outward, the less effective the stretch for your calf.

5. **Take a deep breath in, and as you exhale, gently press your hips forward, keeping your left heel on the ground (see Figure 7-14a).**

6. **Hold the stretch for several deep breaths and then slightly bend your left knee without lifting your heel off the floor (see Figure 7-14b).**

   By bending your knee you stretch an additional muscle in your calf, which is important for ankle flexibility.

7. **Repeat this stretch with your right leg.**

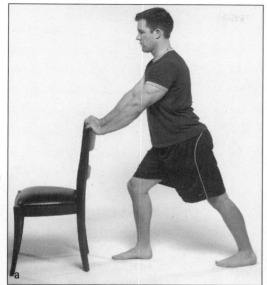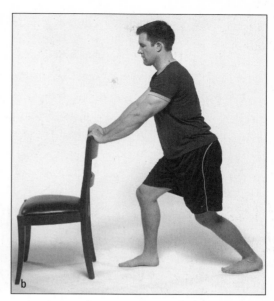

Figure 7-14: Relieving calf pain with the standing calf stretch.

A few do's and don'ts for this exercise:

✔ Do keep your toes and heel in line.

✔ Do keep your heel on the floor.

✔ Do breathe deeply and rhythmically throughout the stretch.

✔ Don't round your back — keep your neck, shoulders, back, hips, and rear leg in one line.

Achilles tendon stretch on one knee

One of the more common severe injuries of the weekend warrior is a torn or ruptured Achilles tendon. This type of injury can only be treated with surgery and/or prolonged immobilization in a cast. Trust me; neither option is any fun at all. Keeping this area flexible and strong is a good preventive approach to keep the injuries and the doctors away. (Who needs apples? Just stretch!)

To do this stretch, follow these steps:

1. **Kneel on one knee with your hips back on your heel and your other foot flat on the floor next to your knee (see Figure 7-15a).**

2. **Place your hands on the floor in front of you and inhale; as you exhale shift your body weight forward, keeping your heel on the floor as you lean forward (see Figure 7-15b).**

   You should feel the stretch in your Achilles tendon in your front leg.

4. **Hold this stretch for 30 seconds or four to five slow, deep breaths.**

5. **Repeat this stretch on your other leg.**

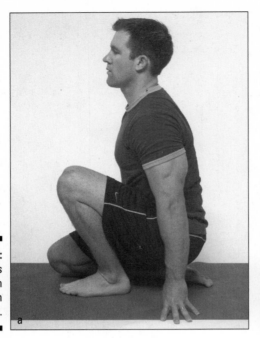 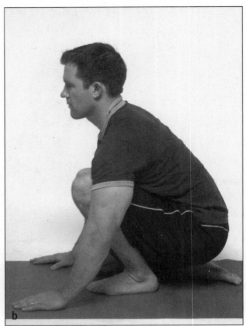

Figure 7-15:
The Achilles tendon stretch on one knee.

A few do's and don'ts for this stretch:

- ✔ Do keep your eyes looking down toward your fingers.
- ✔ Do keep your weight moving forward past your toes.
- ✔ Do keep your hips over your back foot.
- ✔ Don't lift your back heel off the floor.
- ✔ Don't force or bounce the stretch.

Kneeling shin stretch

Probably the most common injury to your shin area is called shin splints. Shin splints happen for many reasons: overuse, working out on a hard surface, fallen arches in your feet, and even lack of flexibility. Try this next stretch to keep this area lengthened and flexible.

Skip this stretch if you have bad knees because the exercise may be uncomfortable for you.

To do this stretch, follow these steps:

1. **Kneel on a carpeted floor or mat with your toes pointed backward.**

2. **Lower your hips and sit on top of your heels (see Figure 7-16a).**

3. **Inhale and as you exhale grab the top of your left foot and gently pull it toward your buttocks (see Figure 7-16b).**

4. **You should feel this stretch in your left shin.**

5. **Hold the stretch for a few seconds and release.**

6. **Repeat this stretch a few more times on your left side and then switch sides, repeating the stretch an equal number of times on the right.**

If this position is uncomfortable or creates pain in your knees because of lack of range of motion, try rolling a towel and placing it behind your knees and under your buttocks. Also, make sure you're on a comfortable mat or carpet while performing this stretch.

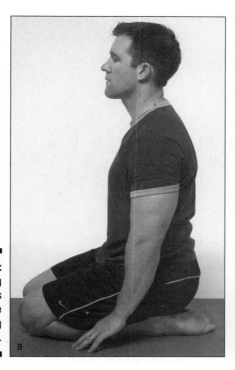 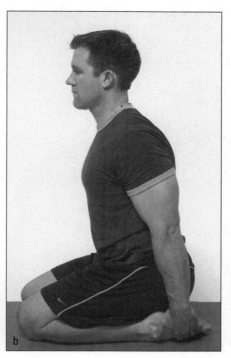

Figure 7-16: Preventing shin splints with the kneeling shin stretch.

A few do's and don'ts for this stretch:

- ✔ Do sit on your heels.
- ✔ Do lift your abdominals while you lift your foot and maintain the natural curve of your spine.
- ✔ Don't allow your buttocks to sit on the floor between your heels — it creates stress on your knees.

On your hands and knees: Bottom of foot stretch

Flexible and limber feet and ankles can absorb the pounding of walking, running, and jumping more efficiently than if your feet and ankles are tight and rigid. This stretch targets the muscles that run along the entire bottom of your feet. It doesn't beat a foot massage, but if you're prone to cramping in your feet you should do this stretch every day.

To do this stretch, follow these steps:

1. **Begin with your hands and knees on the floor (all-fours position).**

2. **Flex your feet so your toes are moving toward your knees (see Figure 7-17a).**

3. **Inhale and gently move your hips back and down toward your heels and move your heels up, toward your hips (see Figure 7-17b).**

   You should feel this stretch on the bottom of your feet.

4. **Hold the stretch for 30 seconds by using deep breathing to help you sink gradually deeper into the stretch.**

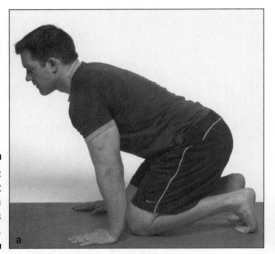 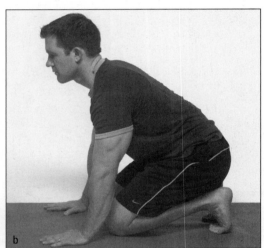

Figure 7-17: A foot stretch in the all-fours position.

A few do's and don'ts for this stretch:

- Do move your hips back toward your heels.
- Do focus on lifting your heels as you gently press the balls of your feet toward the floor.
- Do lift your bellybutton toward your spine.
- Don't hold your breath.

Lying ankle circles

This exercise is designed to loosen up the muscles around your ankles and to increase circulation in your feet and lower legs. To do this exercise, follow these steps:

1. **Lie on your back with your left leg straight out in front of you and your right knee lifted toward your chest.**

2. **Inhale, and as you exhale, circle your right ankle clockwise four to eight times.**

3. **Reverse the circle counterclockwise for four to eight rotations (see Figure 7-18).**

If it's more comfortable, bend your opposite knee while you circle your ankle.

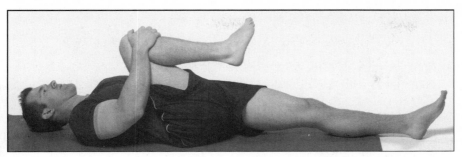

Figure 7-18: Lying ankle circles.

A few do's and don'ts for this exercise:

✔ Do keep your upper back, neck, and shoulders relaxed and tension free while you focus on your ankle.

✔ Do make your ankle circles slow and mindful.

✔ Don't grip your feet or crunch your toes.

In case you always wanted to do the splits

Two kinds of splits — forward splits and straddle or side splits — are both considered advanced stretches because they require extreme flexibility in your hamstrings, hip flexors, quads, and adductors. Keep in mind that doing the splits isn't necessary for everyday life. Gymnasts, cheerleaders, dancers, and advanced athletes in martial arts or figure skating are really the only ones who need that much flexibility. If your goal is to feel better and move more freely, then just stick to the exercises in this chapter.

Is trying to do a split a good idea or a bad idea? For generations, many have regarded achieving a perfect split as the height of flexibility, but because of its allure, it has enticed many people unprepared for the demands of the stretch into an uncomfortable and possibly harmful position. Perhaps the real question isn't whether to attempt the stretch, but why? To do the splits properly requires a real investment of time and discipline, and if you're not performing in Cirque du Soleil, it might not be worth the payoff. Nevertheless, if doing the splits is something you've always wanted to do, follow these guidelines:

1. **Warm up!**

2. **Perform individual stretches for your hamstrings, quads, and inner thighs (see examples in this chapter).**

   Make sure these areas are warm and limber before you make your first attempt.

3. **Begin kneeling on one leg and place your opposite foot out in front of you flat on the floor.**

4. **Slowly slide the knee beneath you backward as far as you can.**

   Notice that your front leg gradually extends. Find your comfort zone and stay there for a few deep breaths.

5. **Inhale and as you exhale, see if you can move the knee back a little farther and take the stretch a little deeper.**

6. **Hold the stretch for 30 seconds and then release the stretch by coming back to the starting position.**

7. **Try the stretch again and repeat two or three times — each time trying to go a little deeper and getting your legs straighter.**

Don't expect to be able to do a perfect split right away. It will take weeks of slowly and progressively increasing your range of motion in the split position. As with any stretch, perform this one slowly and carefully and pay attention to form. In a perfect split, both legs must be straight, both hips must face forward, and the buttock of your front leg should be on the floor. You probably won't get it the first time you try, but you can gradually get a little farther every day. Don't be discouraged.

It's really fun to do something you thought was impossible, and many of you may think it's impossible to do a perfect split. But you never know until you try.

Chapter 8

Total-Body Stretch Routines

In This Chapter

▶ Practicing deep breathing exercises

▶ Performing a ten-minute, total-body routine, using basic stretch exercises

▶ Adding additional stretches when you have more time

In this chapter I've designed a total-body stretching routine that helps teach you body awareness and presents a selection of basic, effective stretches for the entire body in the most accessible, comfortable position possible. The sense of body awareness you develop in this total-body series stays with you always.

If you're just starting a stretching program and this chapter is your first stop, be patient and give yourself time to work up slowly (which means only do what feels comfortable to you). The single most important thing you need to keep in mind when beginning a stretching program is to be *patient*. Rome wasn't built in a day and neither were your muscles — relaxing your tight muscles and getting comfortable with stretching takes longer than a day.

Getting to Your Whole Body in Just Ten Minutes

The total-body routine in this section progresses through three stages:

> ✔ **Breathing** is the most fundamental of all stretching techniques. Breathing helps your muscles relax, which makes your stretches more effective. If your body has any tension, then your muscles won't stretch to their full potential.
>
> ✔ **Correct body alignment** is important for good posture and to prevent injury. The total-body routine helps you find and maintain a neutral spine (keeping your hips, buttocks, and back all in one straight line) to assist in proper alignment. This stretching routine also helps you strengthen your shoulders and upper back so you can stand up tall and proud.
>
> ✔ **Stretching all the major muscle groups** leads to whole-body wellness, and this routine helps you slowly progress through a sequence of stretches designed to concentrate on all those major muscle groups — from your top to the bottom. Just start at the beginning of this routine and work your way through each stretch as prescribed below.

Each stage above is a building block. For instance, after you master the proper technique for breathing, you then use your breath to relax so you can focus on enhanced body awareness throughout the following stretches.

In addition, this total-body routine is full of ACD stretches — Anyone-Can-Do stretches (or at least that's what I call them). This sequence of stretches gently allows you to increase your awareness of your body and the way it feels, while helping you get more comfortable with the basic stretches.

Follow this ten-minute routine every day, and on days you have a little extra time, add the last set of ten stretches, under "When You Just Can't Get Enough: Ten More Minutes of Stretching," later in this chapter, for a comprehensive 20-minute routine.

Deep breathing exercise

The purpose of this simple breathing exercise is to focus on your breathing so when you actually do start stretching, you relax and your muscles are tension free.

If you close your eyes during this exercise you may have more luck clearing your mind of other thoughts. Now is *not* the time to think about what you're having for lunch or whom you may have forgotten to call. This time is for thinking only about your body, your breathing, and your movement.

To do this exercise, follow these steps:

1. **Lie on your back on the floor with your knees bent and your feet flat on the floor.**

   Take a moment to feel neutral spine — the natural curve of your back as you lie on the floor.

2. **Place your hands on your lower abdomen (see Figure 8-1), and inhale deeply through your nose and feel your rib cage expand as you fill your lungs with air.**

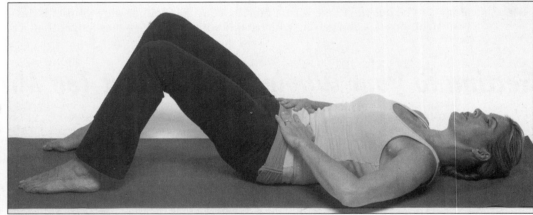

Figure 8-1:
Deep breathing exercise lying on the floor.

3. **As you exhale, push the air out through your nose or mouth.**

   Feel your rib cage shrink back to its original size.

4. **Repeat this exercise five times.**

A few do's and don'ts for this exercise:

✔ Do keep your lower back on the floor during this exercise.

✔ Do keep your body relaxed and free of tension.

✔ Don't forget to feel your rib cage with your hands as it expands and shrinks.

Lying pelvic tilts

This exercise is designed to help you discover body awareness in the hip and pelvis area — which is responsible for many everyday movements like climbing stairs and maintaining your balance. And this stretch not only warms up the muscles around the pelvic girdle but also helps you find and maintain neutral spine.

To do this exercise, follow these steps:

1. **On a comfortable surface such as a carpeted floor or a stretching mat, lie on your back with your knees bent and your feet flat on the floor or mat.**

2. **Inhale deeply and as you exhale, tip your pelvis upward so you feel your lower back gently pressing against the floor (see Figure 8-2a).**

   Keep your upper body relaxed and tension free. Focus on moving only your pelvis.

3. **Release back to neutral spine (see Figure 8-2b).**

4. **Repeat this exercise eight to ten times.**

A few do's and don'ts for this exercise:

- Do keep your upper back on the floor.
- Do keep your neck and shoulders relaxed.
- Don't squeeze your buttocks when you tilt.

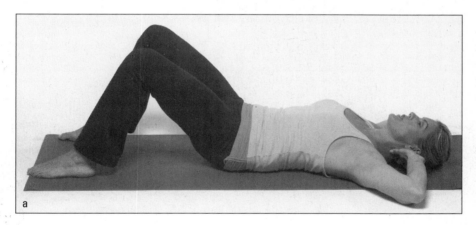

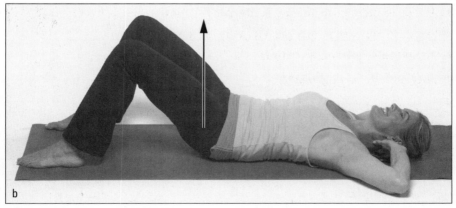

Figure 8-2:
Lying pelvic tilts to warm up your pelvic girdle muscles.

Lying arm circles

The purpose of this exercise is to teach you how to increase body awareness by stabilizing your shoulder girdle (the area surrounding the shoulder) and maintaining neutral spine when you move your arms. This stretch also warms up your shoulders and prepares you for the upper body stretches to come.

To do this exercise, follow these steps:

1. **Lie on your back with your knees bent and your feet flat on the floor with your arms at your sides.**

2. **Take a deep breath and lift your arms above you on the floor (see Figure 8-3a).**

3. **As you exhale, lower your arms back to your sides in a circular pattern as if you were lying in the snow and making a snow angel (see Figure 8-3b).**

4. **Repeat this exercise eight to ten times.**

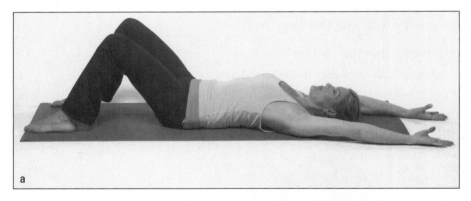

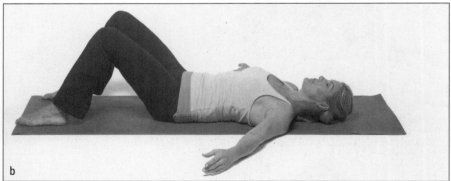

Figure 8-3:
Lying arm
circles.

A few do's and don'ts for this exercise:

✔ Do keep your neck long and relaxed.

✔ Do keep your shoulder blades down as you lift your arms overhead.

✔ Don't arch your back or move your rib cage as you lift your arms.

Lying spinal rotation with bent knees

I love this exercise because it's one of the simplest ways to increase or maintain range of motion in the trunk, hips, and buttocks areas. Flexibility in these areas is crucial for functional fitness — being in shape for everyday life!

To do this exercise, follow these steps:

1. **Lie on your back and bring your knees to your chest and extend your arms out from your sides (see Figure 8-4a).**

2. **Take a deep breath in and as you exhale, slowly lower your legs to one side until they reach the floor, keeping your arms flat on the floor (see in Figure 8-4b).**

   Be sure to keep the opposite shoulder blade and your head on the floor.

3. **Hold this stretch for about 30 seconds, taking several deep breaths as you relax into the stretch.**

4. **Slowly lift your knees back to center and repeat the same stretch on the other side.**

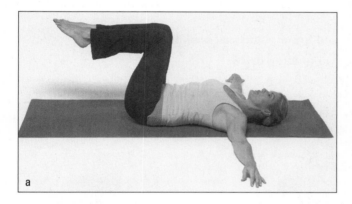

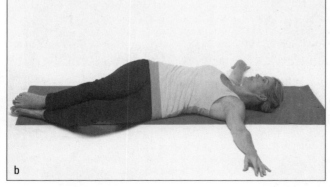

Figure 8-4: Lying spinal rotation for range of motion in your trunk.

Do's and don'ts for this exercise include the following:

✔ Do keep your shoulders down and relaxed.

✔ Don't hold your breath.

Lying neck stretch

This simple stretch is one of the easiest ways to help relieve tension in your neck and shoulders.

You need to be very gentle with this stretch — definitely no forcing the stretch or yanking on your neck.

To do this exercise, follow these steps:

1. **Lie on your back with your knees bent and your feet flat on the floor.**

2. **Interlock your fingers behind your head (see Figure 8-5a).**

3. **Take a deep breath in and as you exhale, slowly lift your head with your hands, bringing your chin toward your chest (see Figure 8-5b).**

   Be sure to keep both shoulder blades on the floor and lift only your neck. Because of where the muscles of your upper back and neck are attached, you diminish the effectiveness of this stretch if you lift your shoulder blades off the floor.

4. **Hold this stretch for about 30 seconds, taking several deep breaths as you relax into the stretch.**

5. **Release the stretch and lower your head back to the floor.**

6. **Repeat this stretch two to three times.**

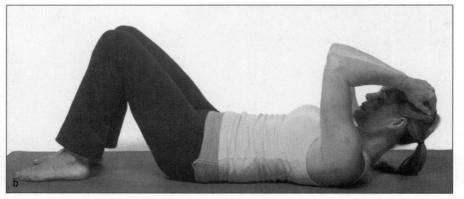

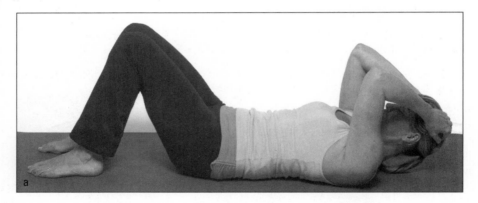

Figure 8-5: Lying neck stretch for releasing neck and shoulder tension.

A few do's and don'ts for this exercise:

✔ Do keep your knees bent and your feet flat on the floor.

✔ Do keep your shoulder blades anchored to the floor and only lift your head.

✔ Don't put too much pressure on your neck with your hands; they should only nudge your head forward.

✔ Don't hold your breath.

Standing hamstring stretch with chair

You feel this stretch in the back of your thighs, which are commonly called your hamstrings. This area is tight for a lot of people, so if you're one of these folks, take your time and really relax into the stretch. Go grab a sturdy chair for this exercise.

To do this exercise, follow these steps:

1. **Stand with your feet about hip-width apart and your hands on the seat of the sturdy chair in front of you.**

2. **Inhale deeply, and hinge from the hips, lowering your upper body toward the chair (see Figure 8-6a).**

3. **Inhale again and as you exhale, try to lower your body even more by bending your elbows (see Figure 8-6b).**

   As you become more flexible, try to lower your elbows to the seat of the chair.

4. **Hold this stretch for 30 seconds.**

   You feel a deeper stretch behind your thighs and in the back of your knees if you keep your back flat and tilt your pelvis toward the ceiling.

5. **Bend your knees and roll your upper body up to a standing position.**

Figure 8-6:
Loosen those tight hamstrings with the standing hamstring stretch and a chair.

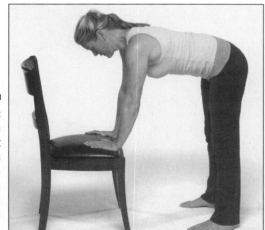
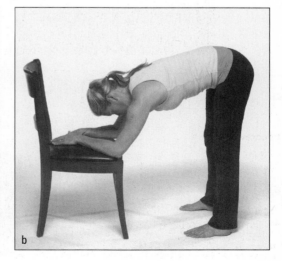

A few do's and don'ts for this exercise:

- Do remember to take several deep breaths during the 30 seconds.
- Do keep your knees straight.
- Don't round your back.
- Don't tuck your hips under.

Standing inner thigh stretch with chair

Although you can stretch your inner thigh area in many different ways, this stretch is probably the easiest way to stretch your groin area without tensing your neck, shoulders, and back.

To do this stretch, follow these steps:

1. **Stand next to a chair.**

2. **Raise your leg that's closest to the chair and place your foot on the seat of the chair.**

   Make sure to keep your hips and shoulders facing forward, as shown in Figure 8-7a.

3. **Exhale slowly as you bend forward and lower your hands toward the floor.**

   Check out Figure 8-7b for the visualization of this stretch. Let gravity do the work for you. If you feel too much strain, place one hand on the seat of the chair to give you a little more control over the stretch.

4. **Gradually deepen the stretch with every exhale as you hold this stretch for 30 seconds.**

   Shake your head "no" to make sure that you aren't holding tension in your neck.

5. **Roll up slowly and repeat the stretch with your other leg.**

Never bounce or force the stretch. This actually can cause the muscles to tighten rather than relax and lengthen.

Figure 8-7: Standing inner thigh stretch with chair.

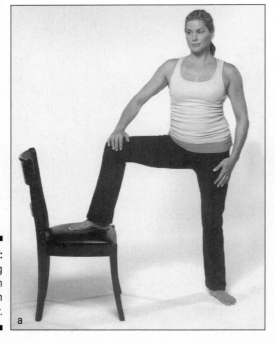
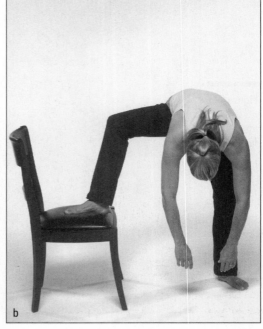

A few do's and don'ts for this stretch:

> ✔ Do tilt your pelvis back so you feel the stretch a little deeper in your groin.
>
> ✔ Do keep your arms and shoulders relaxed and just let gravity gently deepen the stretch.
>
> ✔ Do keep your standing leg straight.
>
> ✔ Don't rush!

Standing quad stretch with support

The front of your thigh is made up of four muscles known as the quadriceps. You probably know them as the "quads." To stretch these muscles, which are important for climbing stairs and lifting heavy things, follow these steps:

1. **Stand up tall with your right hand on a sturdy chair or wall.**

2. **Bend your left knee and raise your heel toward your buttocks.**

3. **Reach with your left hand and grab hold of your heel (see Figure 8-8a).**

4. **Inhale deeply and as you exhale, slowly lower your bent knee until it is even or side by side with your other knee (see Figure 8-8b).**

   Try to keep the inside of your thighs touching and focus on moving your knee back, not forcing your foot to touch your buttocks. To really feel this stretch correctly, try to tuck your pelvis under and think about your tailbone moving toward the floor.

5. **Hold this stretch for 30 seconds or about four to five slow, deep breaths.**

6. **Repeat the same stretch on your right leg.**

To make this stretch more challenging, let go of the chair or wall and you'll be improving your balance while you stretch your quads.

Figure 8-8:
Standing quad stretch with support.

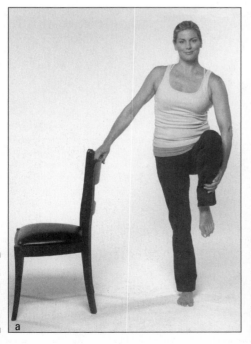
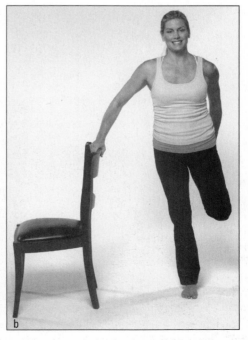

A few do's and don't for this stretch:

- ✔ Do stand up tall with good posture.
- ✔ Do keep your standing knee slightly bent
- ✔ Don't compress your knee by pulling your heel to your buttock.
- ✔ Don't pull your heel to the outside of your hip.

Standing chest stretch

This simple chest stretch can be done anywhere and should be done several times a day, especially if you find yourself sitting a lot. It helps keep your chest muscles from tightening up and can prevent that hunched-over look.

To do this stretch, follow these steps:

1. **Stand up tall and clasp your hands together by your buttocks and behind your back (see Figure 8-9a).**

   If you have difficulty getting your hands together behind your back, try holding the end of a small towel in each hand.

2. **Take a deep breath and as you exhale, gently straighten your arms and lift your hands up toward the ceiling and away from your back (see Figure 8-9b).**

   Lift as high as you can while still standing tall. Be sure not to bend over.

3. **Hold this stretch for 30 seconds.**

Figure 8-9:
Standing
chest
stretch.

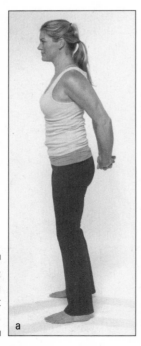
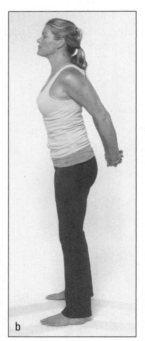

a   b

A few do's and don'ts for this stretch:

✔ Do stand up tall with good posture.

✔ Do keep your knees slightly bent.

✔ Don't tense or lift your shoulders.

✔ Don't hold your breath.

When You Just Can't Get Enough: Ten More Minutes of Stretching

When you get comfortable with the stretches in the previous sections and you have a little more time, try adding on a few more stretches from this section to make a comprehensive 20-minute routine.

Seated buttocks and hip stretch

This stretch can be done in different positions, but I think it's best that you sit for this stretch. It's the most comfortable way to stretch this area and the easiest position to get into if your muscles are very tight.

This stretch is a good one to try if you have sciatic pain. I talk more about sciatic pain in Chapter 6 and 7.

To do this stretch, follow these steps:

1. **Sit on a chair with one leg crossed over the other and let your ankle rest on your thigh.**

2. **Place your elbow on the inside of your knee and inhale.**

3. **As you exhale, lean forward, lengthen your spine, and tilt your pelvis back (see Figure 8-10).**

4. **Hold the stretch for 30 seconds, gradually deepening the stretch on every exhale.**

5. **Repeat the stretch on the other side.**

A few do's and don'ts for this stretch:

✔ Do keep your shoulder blades down.

✔ Do keep your chest lifted.

✔ Do be patient and let the stretch deepen with each breath.

✔ Don't lift one hip or lean to one side.

✔ Don't bounce or jerk.

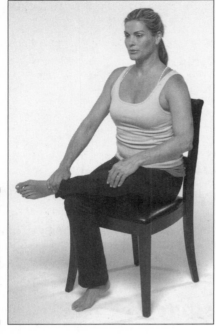

Figure 8-10: Seated buttocks and hip stretch that really helps relieve sciatic pain.

Seated foot and ankle stretches

These next three stretches are for the muscles that surround your ankle and foot.

It's not a bad idea to do ankle circles in both directions several times during the day (see Chapter 7 for an ankle circle exercise). Whether you sit all day or stand all day, this stretch brings better circulation and warmth to your ankles and feet and keeps this area flexible. If the muscles around your ankles are inflexible, you're at a higher risk of injuring your ankle.

To do these stretches, follow these steps:

1. **Sit up very tall in a chair with your left leg crossed over your right knee and your ankle resting on your thigh.**

2. **Hold on to the top of your foot with your right hand and your ankle with your left hand.**

3. **Gently pull back on your foot (kind of like pointing your toes).**

   See Figure 8-11a. You should feel the stretch in the top of your foot.

4. **Hold the stretch for 30 seconds and then release.**

5. **Now, grab your toes with your left hand and your heel with your right hand and gradually pull your toes back toward your shin.**

   See Figure 8-11b. You should feel this stretch in the bottom of your foot.

6. **Hold this stretch for 30 seconds and then release.**

7. **Grab your ankle with your left hand and reach your right hand underneath your foot and grab hold of the top of your foot.**

8. **Gently pull your foot toward the ceiling, and turn it as if you were looking for something on the bottom of your foot.**

   See Figure 8-11c. You should feel the stretch on the outside of your ankle.

9. **Hold the stretch for 30 seconds and then release.**

10. **Repeat the same stretches on your right foot and ankle.**

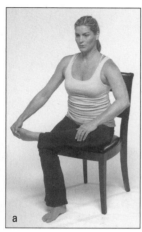 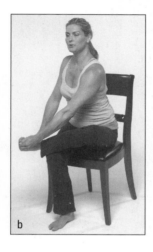 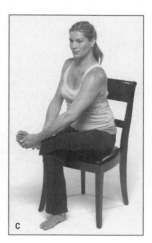

Figure 8-11: Seated foot and ankle stretches.

A few do's and don'ts for this stretch:

- ✔ Do keep your chest lifted and your spine very tall.
- ✔ Do relax and breathe.
- ✔ Don't lift one hip or lean to one side.
- ✔ Don't force or pulse the stretches.

Seated triceps stretch with side reach

You feel this stretch in the back of your upper arms and mid-back too. To do this stretch, follow these steps:

1. **Sit up very tall with your right arm overhead and elbow bent behind you so the tips of your fingers are touching the back of your shoulder.**

2. **Place your left hand on your raised elbow (see Figure 8-12a).**

3. **Take a deep breath in, and as you exhale begin to gently pull your right elbow behind your head, reaching your right fingers down your back toward your spine (see Figure 8-12b).**

4. **Take another deep breath in and as you exhale, lean to the left as far as feels comfortable, being careful not to twist.**

5. **Hold this stretch for about 30 seconds and then come back to center and gently release your arm.**

6. **Give your arms a little shake and repeat the stretch with the left arm.**

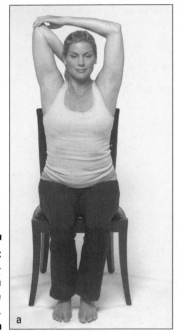 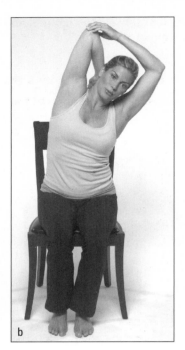

Figure 8-12:
Seated tri-
ceps stretch
with side
reach.

A few do's and don't for this stretch:

✔ Do sit up tall with good posture.

✔ Do keep your shoulders facing the front.

✔ Don't tense or lift your shoulders.

✔ Don't hold your breath.

✔ Don't arch your back or open your rib cage.

✔ Don't jam or force your elbow back.

Seated lateral shoulder stretch

This stretch is for the middle part of your deltoid muscle. If you're wondering if you even have a deltoid, the answer is yes — it's the muscle that runs across the front, middle, and back of your shoulder.

To do this stretch, shown in Figure 8-13, follow the steps below:

1. **Sit up very tall and raise your right elbow to shoulder height and place your right hand on your left shoulder.**

2. **Place your left hand on your right elbow and as you exhale, gently pull your elbow toward your left shoulder.**

3. **Hold this stretch for 30 seconds and then repeat the steps with your left arm.**

If you want to try a slightly different version of the same stretch, try keeping your arm straight, rather than bending at the elbow, as you reach across your body.

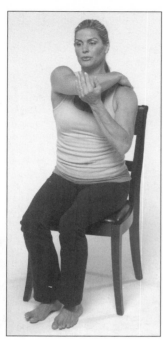

Figure 8-13: Seated lateral shoulder stretch.

A few do's and don't for this stretch:

- ✔ Do sit up tall with good posture.
- ✔ Do keep your hips and shoulders facing the front of the room.
- ✔ Do keep your shoulder blade down.
- ✔ Don't twist at the waist.
- ✔ Don't tense or lift your shoulders.
- ✔ Don't hold your breath.
- ✔ Don't jam or force your elbow back.

Seated forward bend

You should feel this stretch along your spine and throughout your entire back. By hinging at your hips, you release any tension in your back muscles and help stretch out the vertebrae in your spine.

To do this stretch, follow these steps:

1. **Sit on a chair with your feet flat on the floor and your tummy pulled in or abdominals tight (see Figure 8-14a).**

2. **Inhale and as you exhale, bend forward at the hips as far as you can comfortably stretch, letting your arms hang down toward the ground (see Figure 8-14b).**

3. **Hold the stretch for 30 seconds or four to five slow, deep breaths.**

4. **Slowly roll back up, stacking one vertebra on top of the other until you're sitting up tall.**

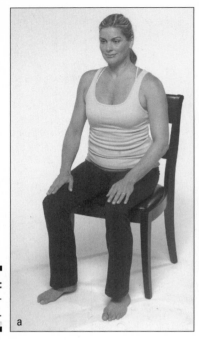 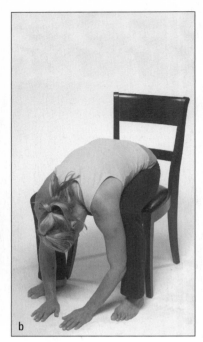

Figure 8-14: Seated forward bend.

A few do's and don't for this stretch:

- Do start the motion from your hips, not from your back.
- Do start the stretch in the comfort zone, gradually getting deeper with each breath.
- Don't hold your breath.
- Don't force the stretch.
- Don't hold tension in your shoulders.

Standing wrist stretch

This stretch increases and maintains flexibility in your wrists and forearms. To do this stretch, follow these steps:

1. **Stand tall with your feet hip-width apart.**

2. **Hold your arms straight and lift them slightly out in front of your body, your hands at about the level of your hips, palms facing each other (see Figure 8-15a).**

3. **As you exhale, rotate your thumbs downward as if you were turning two knob handles (see Figure 8-15b).**

4. **Continue rotating as far as you can for about 30 seconds.**

It may be more comfortable for you to hold this stretch for a few seconds and then repeat several times instead of just holding for the full 30 seconds.

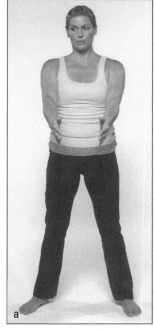 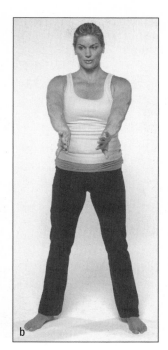

Figure 8-15:
Standing
wrist
stretch —
stand up tall
and rotate
your wrists
inward.

A few do's and don't for this stretch:

✔ Do stand up tall with good posture.

✔ Do keep your elbows slightly bent.

✔ Don't tense or lift your shoulders.

✔ Don't hold your breath.

✔ Don't lock your elbows.

Standing forearm stretch

This stretch helps combat the discomfort caused by repetitive stress injuries like carpal tunnel syndrome. You should feel this stretch throughout your forearms and wrists.

To do this stretch, follow these steps:

1. **Stand up tall with the palm of one hand against the fingers of the other hand.**

   Keep your elbows lifted toward the ceiling.

2. **Inhale and as you exhale gently press the heel of your hand against your fingers (see Figure 8-16).**

3. **Hold this stretch for 30 seconds.**

4. **Repeat on the other hand.**

If this stretch is more comfortable to hold for a few seconds and then repeat several times instead of just holding for the full 30 seconds, that's okay. Do what makes you comfortable. Stretching shouldn't be painful!

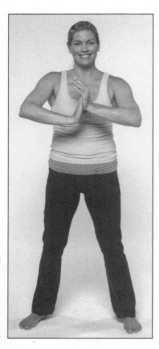

Figure 8-16:
Standing
forearm
stretch.

A few do's and don't for this stretch:

- ✔ Do stand up tall with good posture.
- ✔ Don't tense or lift your shoulders.
- ✔ Don't hold your breath.
- ✔ Don't let your elbows drop.

Standing side reach

Finishing this routine with a good side reach gets you geared up for more complex, integrated stretches that you do later on. You feel this stretch in your shoulder, back, abs, and even the top part of your hip.

To do this stretch, follow these steps:

1. **Stand up very tall with your feet apart and toes forward.**

2. **Reach your left arm directly overhead, using the muscles in your upper back to keep your shoulder blade down.**

3. **Inhale and as you exhale, bend to the right and reach with your left arm up and out and away from your body.**

   Make sure to keep your hips and legs anchored to the floor. Rest your right hand on your right thigh for extra support (see Figure 8-17).

4. **Hold this stretch for 30 seconds or four to five slow, deep breaths.**

5. **Repeat the stretch on your other side.**

If you notice tension in your shoulders, just keep your elbow bent instead of reaching with a straight arm.

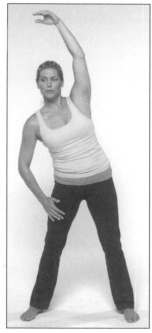

Figure 8-17: The standing side reach that stretches your abs, back, and shoulders.

A few do's and don't for this stretch:

- ✔ Do bend only to the side — no twisting or arching your back.
- ✔ Do keep your shoulder blades down.
- ✔ Do open up your chest, keeping your shoulders and hips facing forward.
- ✔ Do breathe through the stretch.
- ✔ Don't hold the stretch if you feel tension or pain.
- ✔ Don't arch your back or bend forward.
- ✔ Don't twist.
- ✔ Don't lift your opposite heel; keep both feet flat on the floor.

Part III

From the Daily Grind to Ways to Unwind: Routines to Fit Your Life and Needs

The 5th Wave   By Rich Tennant

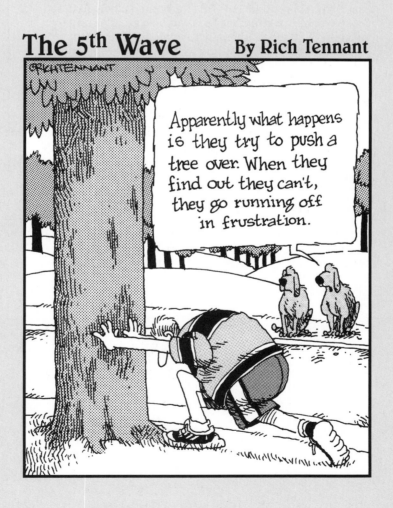

Apparently what happens is they try to push a tree over. When they find out they can't, they go running off in frustration.

In this part . . .

I give you specific stretches for specific situations. For instance, in Chapter 9, you find three routines for three different times of the day. For the morning, I recommend my AM routine. For the afternoon, I clue you in to some wonderful stretches that can be a great alternative to a cup of coffee. And finally the chapter ends with a quiet and calming PM routine to help you unwind and relax after a busy and hectic day (and help you get some sleep, I hope!).

In Chapter 10, you discover stretch routines to help you make it through your workday. If you've been cooped up on an airplane, trapped in a car, or chained to your desk, this chapter is for you. These stretches help get you up and out of your seat to aid circulation and prevent muscle tension. If for some reason you need to remain seated all day (for instance, you have a stickler for a boss), I provide a routine that you can do in your chair.

Chapter 11 features routines for warming up and cooling down. And finally, Chapter 12 is geared for the weekend warrior, featuring specific stretches for specific sports to help improve your performance and enhance your range of motion.

Chapter 9

When the Cock Crows and the Evening Wind Blows: AM/PM Stretch Routines

*I*t's true that stretching first thing in the morning can wake you up and get you energized, while stretching at the end of the day helps you relax and wind down. And there are specific stretches that I recommend in this chapter for the morning and for the evening. However, the key ingredient in making any stretching program work is its *intention*. Stretching in the morning gives you time to feel your body waking up and to focus on your day; stretching in the evening allows you to concentrate on yourself and gently work out your tensions from the day. In both instances, stretching is a tool that allows you to take care of yourself in the way you need most — at that moment.

Nothing is going to make you younger, but stretching definitely makes you *feel* younger! The best way to get that youthful feeling is to stretch every day. Ideally you should be able to find structured time for your flexibility training, such as stretching after your workout or taking yoga or stretching classes regularly. But that's not always possible, so on days when life gets in the way, you have to grab a moment for yourself here and there. First thing in the morning or the last thing at night are perfect times to steal a little interlude for yourself. Remember, it's the little things in life that matter, and doing a little something every day goes a long way toward keeping your body flexible, pain free, and feeling young.

In this chapter, you get a terrific series of stretches to help release any built-up tension in your lower back muscles and loosen up your upper body. I also give you a series of energizing stretches to help get you going right around midday when everyone can use a pick-me-up (and I'm not talking coffee, either!).

A Good Excuse to Stay in Bed: Stretches to Start the Day

I'm not promising if you do these next few stretches every day before you get out of bed that you'll bounce out of bed like my 4-year-old Bella does every morning (yikes!), but I do promise you less morning stiffness and that your blood will actually be pumping *before* you have that first cup of coffee.

Most of the stretches in the AM routine are to be done before you get out of bed. The goal of these stretches is to loosen up your joints and get your muscles lengthened after moving so little for so long while sleeping. Make sure to keep your copy of this book on your nightstand (or under your pillow)!

Supine alternating knee to chest

This exercise is designed to help you slowly begin to stretch your lower back and hamstrings while loosening the muscles around your hips.

First thing in the morning your joints are stiff and your muscles are tight, so make sure that you do this stretch gently and progressively, rhythmically and slowly. The last thing you want to do as soon as you wake up is tear your muscle fibers and *cause* aches and pains.

Doing this exercise first with both knees bent allows a little more time for your back to warm up properly.

To do this exercise, follow these steps:

1. **Lie on your back with your knees bent and your feet flat on the bed.**

2. **Inhale deeply and as you exhale, lift your left knee toward your chest, using your hands for guidance (see Figure 9-1).**

   Don't hold the top of your kneecap. This can cause pressure on your knee joint. Instead, place your hands under your knee as you guide your knee forward.

3. **Hold the stretch for 30 seconds or four to five slow, deep breaths and then release.**

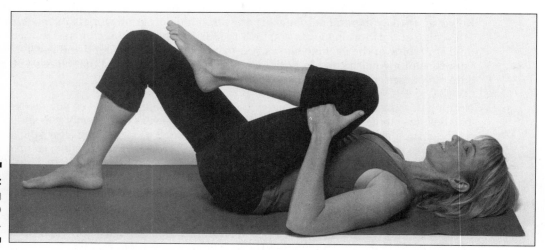

Figure 9-1: Alternating knees to chest.

4. **Lower your leg back to the beginning position and repeat on your right leg.**

5. **Alternate left and right legs for eight to ten repetitions and then extend both legs straight.**

6. **Keeping your left leg straight, bring your right knee toward your chest, using your hands for guidance (see Figure 9-2).**

   Try to bring your knee a little closer to your chest than when you had both knees bent at the beginning of this stretch. Remember not to hold the top of your kneecap. Instead, place your hands under your knee as you guide your knee forward.

7. **Hold the stretch for 30 seconds or four to five slow, deep breaths.**

8. **Lower your knee back to the extended position and repeat on your left leg.**

9. **Repeat this exercise for eight to ten repetitions.**

A few do's and don'ts for this exercise:

✔ Do exhale as you bring your knee forward.

✔ Do keep your neck and shoulders relaxed.

✔ Don't bring your knee so far forward that it causes your hips to lift off your bed.

✔ Don't hold the top of your kneecap.

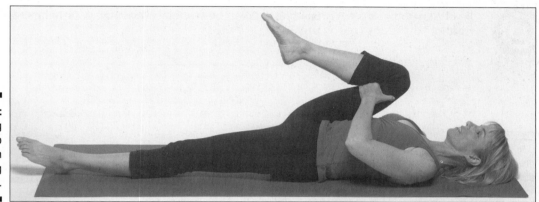

Figure 9-2:
Alternating knee to chest with one leg straight.

Both knees to chest

This stretch is my all-time favorite for my lower back. The movements are gentle and simple, so I think it's the perfect way to wake up my lower back. I hope you think so, too!

To do this exercise, follow these steps:

1. **Lie on your back with your knees bent and your feet flat on the bed.**

2. **Bring both knees toward your chest, placing your hands under each knee for support.**

   Breathe deeply. See Figure 9-3 for placement of your knees and hands. Everyone has different body types. To make this stretch comfortable, you may have to adjust where you put your knees. Some people will be more comfortable with their knees wide; some people might feel the stretch more with their knees closer to their chest. Move your knees around a little to find the spot that's most comfortable for you and allows you to breathe easily.

3. **Hold the stretch for 30 seconds or four to five slow, deep breaths.**

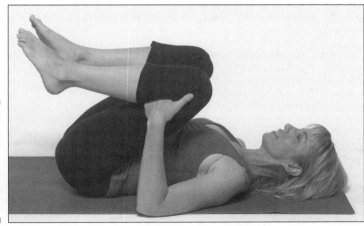

Figure 9-3:
Bringing your knees to your chest to stretch the lower back.

A few do's and don'ts for this exercise:

- ✔ Do breath slowly and rhythmically.
- ✔ Do keep your hands under your knees to prevent any undue pressure on your knees.
- ✔ Don't lift your hips off the bed; try to maintain neutral spine.

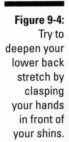

If your lower back is fairly flexible, deepen the stretch by clasping your hands together in front of your shins (see Figure 9-4).

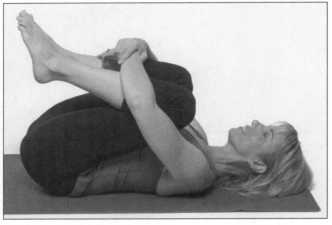

Figure 9-4:
Try to deepen your lower back stretch by clasping your hands in front of your shins.

Spinal rotation with bent knees

This exercise lengthens and stretches the muscles of your back and abdominals. Use a pillow to soften the stretch for the morning. This stretch is great to get you ready for your day!

To do this exercise, follow these steps:

1. **Lie on your back with your knees bent and your feet flat on the bed.**
2. **Bring both knees toward your chest, placing your hands under each knee for support.**
3. **Take a deep breath in, and as you exhale, release your hands from your knees and slowly lower your legs to one side.**
4. **Extend the arm on the opposite side straight out to your side (see Figure 9-5).**
5. **Hold this stretch for 30 seconds, taking several deep breaths as you relax into the stretch.**
6. **Slowly lift your knees back to center and repeat the same stretch on the other side.**

A few do's and don'ts for this exercise:

- ✔ Do keep your knees at a right angle.
- ✔ Do keep your shoulders down and relaxed.
- ✔ Don't hold your breath.

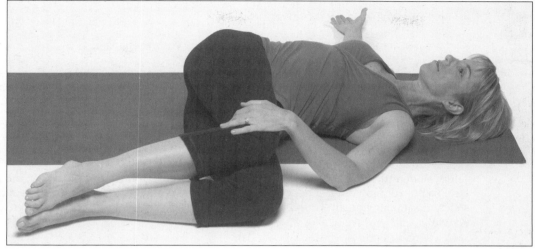

Figure 9-5:
Performing the spinal rotation with bent knees.

Total body stretch

When you wake up in the morning, do you stretch your body either before you get up or after you stand up? Sometimes, nothing feels better than stretching out those sleepy muscles! This stretch may be common sense, but most people need a good reminder of how to stretch the whole body correctly and most effectively. ***Note:*** Breathing is key.

To do this exercise, follow these steps:

1. **Lie on your back with your arms extended over your head.**

2. **Inhale deeply and stretch your arms and your legs as far as you can in opposite directions (see Figure 9-6).**

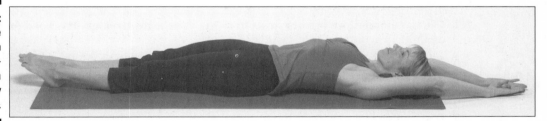

Figure 9-6:
Lying on the floor with arms over-head for a full body stretch.

3. **As you exhale, release the stretch and relax your whole body.**

4. **Repeat this exercise three or four times, each time trying to reach and stretch a little farther.**

   Pull your bellybutton toward your spine as you stretch and lengthen.

5. **After a few repetitions, try reaching one side at a time.**

   As you inhale, reach and stretch your right side only. Exhale and relax; repeat on your left side.

A few do's and don'ts for this exercise:

✔ Do point your toes and lengthen your legs as you reach.

✔ Don't arch your back.

✔ Don't hold your breath.

A Midafternoon Pick-Me-Up

There's no getting around the fact that three in the afternoon is a low point in most people's day. You're running out of energy and fighting off sleep. So the next time you feel like taking a siesta or making an afternoon run for an emergency cappuccino, try an energizing stretch instead!

Overhead forward arm swings

A very important part of overall fitness is being able to maintain your balance. Not only will this rhythmic full-body stretch wake you up, energize you, and lengthen your spine, but also it can help improve your balance, which means less accidents throughout the day when you're climbing stairs or carrying groceries or your kids.

To do this exercise, follow these steps:

1. **Stand tall with your feet together and your arms to your sides.**

2. **Inhale and reach your arms overhead, while raising your heels off the floor so you balance on the balls of your feet (see Figure 9-7a).**

   Hold the pose for a count of three as you maintain your balance.

3. **As you exhale, let your arms swing down as you bend your knees and shift your weight to your heels (see Figure 9-7b).**

4. **Use the momentum of your arms to swing your arms back up overhead and balance again.**

   If you're having trouble balancing at the top of this exercise, check to make sure that your abdominals are pulled in and your shoulders are pressed down.

5. **Exhale and lower again.**

6. **Repeat this exercise five times.**

   On the last one, hold the balance for as long as you can.

A few do's and don'ts for this exercise:

✔ Do keep your abdominals lifted.

✔ Do keep your shoulder blades down, especially when you raise your arms overhead.

✔ Do think of your spine getting longer each time you reach up.

✔ Don't let your belly stick out or compress your lower back.

✔ Don't hold your arms up behind your shoulders.

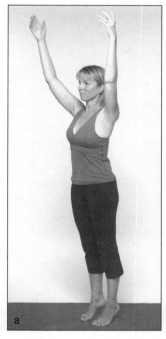
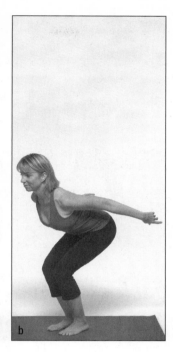

Figure 9-7: Overhead forward swings.

Standing spinal twist with overhead reach

This stretch gets circulation back into your spine, especially if you've been inactive for a while. It's the perfect stretch to get you moving again.

To do this stretch, follow these steps:

1. **Stand tall with your feet apart, your abs and chest lifted, your shoulders back and down, and your arms to your sides (see Figure 9-8a).**

   Keep your feet wide and your knees bent. This position keeps your center of gravity low and makes it easier to keep your upper body relaxed.

2. **Inhale and as you exhale, bend your knees and pivot on your left big toe, turning your hips and shoulders to the right as you reach your left arm overhead (see Figure 9-8b).**

3. **Repeat on the left side (see Figure 9-8c).**

4. **Repeat the stretch for 16 to 20 repetitions, keeping your movement controlled and relaxed.**

A few do's and don'ts for this stretch:

- ✔ Do keep your knees bent at all times.
- ✔ Do keep your abdominals lifted.
- ✔ Do turn your hips all the way to the side.
- ✔ Don't force or jerk the movement — it should flow from side to side.
- ✔ Don't lock your knees.

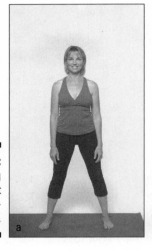
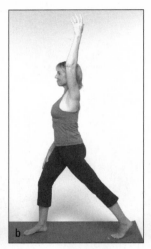
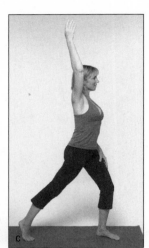

Figure 9-8:
Standing spinal twist with overhead reach.

Lengthening back extension

The purpose of this stretch is to bring circulation to the muscles along your spine. If you have poor posture, or you've been sitting for an extended period of time, you probably have been rounding your back and slouching, which zaps your body of energy. This stretch straightens and lengthens your spine, which is great for improving mobility of your back.

To do this stretch, follow these steps:

1. **Lie on your belly with your palms on the floor next to your chest with your elbows bent and your legs straight and together.**

   Make sure to keep your neck in line with the rest of your spine (see Figure 9-9a).

2. **Inhale and as you exhale, lengthen your spine, lift your chest, and begin to straighten your elbows as you push up with your arms** (see Figure 9-9b).

   Keep your elbows close to your sides and squeeze your buttocks tightly to prevent undo compression of your spine. Imagine the space between each vertebra increasing, lengthening your spine.

3. **Hold the stretch for a few seconds (or as long as it's comfortable) and then slowly lower your body down to the starting position.**

4. **Repeat two or three more times.**

A few do's and don'ts for this stretch:

- ✔ Do keep your neck long and in line with the rest of your spine.
- ✔ Do keep your shoulder blades down.
- ✔ Do pull your belly in toward your spine.
- ✔ Do squeeze your buttocks tightly to prevent pressure in your lower back.
- ✔ Don't compress your lower back.

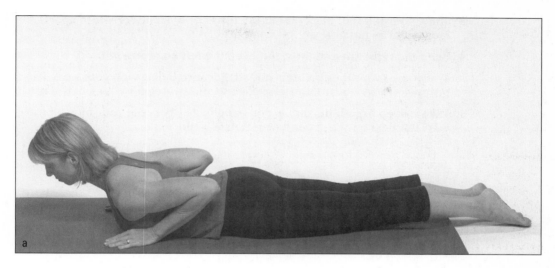

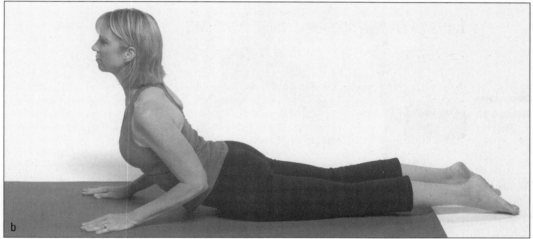

Figure 9-9:
Back exten-
sion and
energizer.

Winding Down before Heading for Dreamland

If you have a difficult time unwinding before bed (and who doesn't?), a few stretches may be just the thing for you. Try these next few stretches after you're ready for bed.

Standing calf stretch

This stretch is great for anyone who has to stand for extended periods of time at work during the day. Stretching your calf muscles before bed helps prevent leg cramps that can happen during the night.

To do this exercise, follow these steps:

1. **Face your bed, and stand an inch or two away from your bed with your feet together.**

2. **Bend forward and place your hands directly in front of you on your bed.**

3. **Move your left foot back (about the distance of shoulder-width apart), keeping your foot as flat as possible on the floor.**

4. **Bend the right knee slightly, but keep the left knee straight.**

   Try to keep your toes pointing directly forward in line with your heel. The more you turn your toes outward, the less effective the stretch for your calf will be.

5. **Take a deep breath in, and as you exhale, gently press your hips forward, keeping your left heel on the ground (see Figure 9-10).**

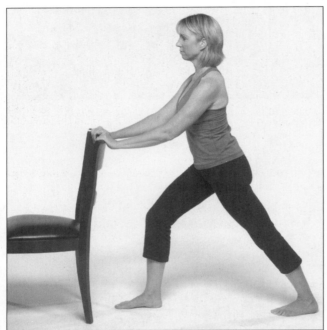

Figure 9-10: Use your bed as a support when you do the standing calf stretch.

6. **Hold the stretch for several deep breaths.**

7. **Slightly bend your left knee without lifting your heel off the floor.**

   By bending your knee you stretch an additional muscle in your calf, which is important for ankle flexibility.

8. **Repeat this stretch on your right leg.**

A few do's and don'ts for this exercise:

  ✔ Do keep your toes and heel in line.

  ✔ Do keep your heel on the floor.

  ✔ Do breathe deeply and rhythmically throughout the stretch.

  ✔ Don't round your back. Try to keep your back straight and press your hips forward.

Lying hip opener

Now it's time to get in bed. This stretch opens up your hips, which is great for a better night's sleep because your tight groin muscles loosen up.

To do this exercise, follow these steps:

1. **Lie on your back with your knees bent and the soles of your feet touching each other (see Figure 9-11).**

   Make sure that your feet are at a comfortable distance from your hips. If your back is arching, your feet are probably too close to your hips.

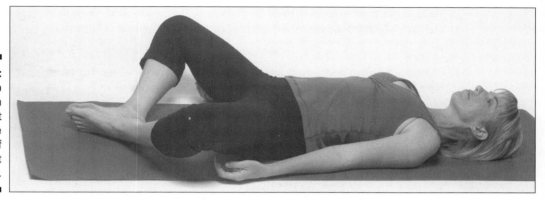

Figure 9-11:
Lying hip opener with knees bent and the soles of your feet together.

2. **Inhale deeply and as you exhale, relax your legs and let gravity gently pull your knees toward the bed.**

   Everybody is different, and your knees may not move too close to the bed. As long as you feel a gentle stretch along the inner thighs, and no pain in your lower back, you're doing fine.

3. **Hold this stretch for 30 seconds or four to five slow, deep breaths.**

A few do's and don'ts for this exercise:

- Do remember to take several deep breaths during the 30 seconds.
- Don't bounce your knees downward or try to force your knees toward the bed.
- Don't arch your back.

Massaging your dogs when they start barkin'

Very few things in life are more relaxing then a foot massage. Unfortunately, you may not have a licensed masseuse at your beck and call, so you have to take things into your own hands.

To do this exercise, follow these steps:

1. **Sit comfortably on the side of your bed and wiggle your toes and circle your ankles a few times.**

   This action increases circulation and helps relax the muscles of your ankles and feet.

2. **Place your right ankle on your left thigh.**

3. **Place your thumbs on the pads of your toes and make circular motions, using medium pressure.**

4. **After circling a few times on each toe, move down to the root or base of your toes, continually applying medium pressure with each circular motion.**

5. **Continue the circular motion across the width of the ball of your foot.**

6. **Move down in a zigzag pattern across the entire length of your foot.**

   Try to massage every spot of the sole of your foot, from your toes to your heel.

7. **End by gently stroking the sole of your foot from top to bottom.**

8. **Repeat the massage on your left foot.**

You may need to use a little more pressure around your heel and ankle. If your feet need a little extra attention, try doing the foot and ankle stretches in Chapter 8.

Lying stretch to take a load off neck and shoulders

This stretch focuses on your neck and shoulders and helps relieve any stress you may have accumulated over the day. To do this stretch, follow these steps:

1. **Lie on your back in your bed with your knees bent and feet flat on your bed.**

2. **Place your hands on the back of your head and point your elbows toward the ceiling.**

3. **Exhale and slowly lift your head while keeping your shoulder blades on your bed (see Figure 9-12).**

   You should feel this stretch in the back of your neck and shoulders.

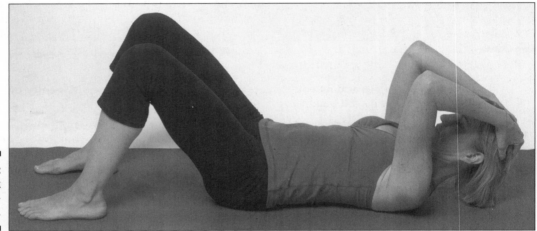

Figure 9-12: Lying neck and shoulder stretch.

4. **Hold this stretch for 30 seconds and then release by slowly lowering your head back to your pillow.**

5. **Repeat this stretch a few times or whatever feels most comfortable to you.**

 Never bounce or force this stretch. Be careful not to jam your chin into your chest, which could cause you to overstretch your neck muscles.

 A few do's and don'ts for this stretch:

- ✔ Do hold your hands at the base of your head and top of your neck.
- ✔ Do keep your body relaxed and your shoulders down.
- ✔ Don't lift your shoulder blades off the bed.
- ✔ Don't hold your breath!

Lying buttocks and hip stretch with legs crossed

This stretch is really good to do if you've been sitting all day and feel tight in your lower body and legs. I also love this stretch for stretching out the lower back by bringing in your knees toward your chest.

To do this stretch, follow these steps:

1. **Lie on your back in your bed with your knees bent and feet flat on your bed.**

2. **Lift your left foot and place the outside of your left ankle on your right thigh, just above your knee.**

3. **Raise your right foot off the bed and bring your knee toward your chest (see Figure 9-13a).**

4. **Interlock your fingers behind your knee.**

5. **Inhale and as you exhale, gently pull your right knee closer to your chest with your hands.**

6. **With your left elbow, gently press your left knee away from you (see Figure 9-13b).**

7. **Hold the stretch for 30 seconds, gradually deepening the stretch with every exhale.**

8. **Repeat the stretch with your right foot on your left thigh.**

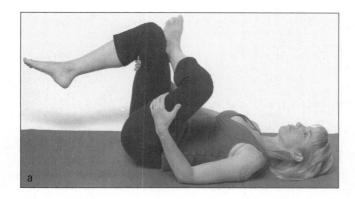

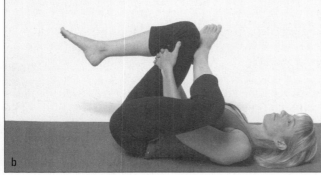

Figure 9-13:
Lying but-
tocks and
hip stretch
with legs
crossed.

A few do's and don'ts for this stretch:

✔ Do keep your shoulder blades down and your upper body relaxed.

✔ Do be patient and let the stretch deepen with each breath.

✔ Don't lift your hips off the bed or lean to one side.

Chapter 10

Stretching Out the Workday: Stretches for Work and for the Road

. . . .

In This Chapter

▶ Stretching as part of your work and travel day
▶ Performing stretches while sitting at your desk
▶ Stretching on the move

. . . .

*Y*our bodies weren't designed to sit for hours at a time. Do you think the cave men would've survived if they had sat still all day? No, they would've been a buffet lunch for some hungry T-Rex. But nowadays, no one has to run from giant carnivores every day. As a matter of fact, in the last 50 years, our lifestyles have changed so dramatically that we've developed an entirely new set of problems because of it: stress headaches, low back pain, muscular tightness and imbalance, repetitive stress injuries, such as carpal tunnel syndrome, and the special selection of aches and pains brought on by the ordeal of modern travel.

This chapter is composed of two sections — one that shows you exercises to do away from your desk (or confined space) to combat the constricting effects of sitting for long periods of time and another series of stretches for when you must stay sitting. Either way, these exercises go a long way toward helping your work and travel lives evolve into healthier, more comfortable forms of existence.

Get Off Your Buttocks!

Whether you're a student, a traveler, a computer jockey, or couch potato, there comes a time when you tend to sit for way too long. Sitting too long on a regular basis can, over time, shorten your hip flexors and the muscles in your hamstrings, chest, and back, resulting in uncomfortable muscle tension.

 Experts recommend getting up out of your chair a couple of times an hour, or more specifically, taking 3- to 5-minute breaks every 20 to 40 minutes. Whenever you get up from your desk at work, or if you get a chance to stretch your legs during a plane flight, choose from the following selections of stretching exercises to help lengthen your muscles, reduce stress and tension, and get your blood pumping again — and in turn, sitting still will feel a lot less like hard work.

Standing chest stretch

This simple chest stretch should be done several times a day, especially if you find yourself sitting a lot. The stretch can actually be done anywhere, and it helps keep your chest muscles from tightening and shortening, which prevents that hunched-over look.

To do this stretch, follow these steps:

1. **Stand up tall and clasp your hands together behind your back just above your tailbone (see Figure 10-1a).**

   If you have difficulty getting your hands together behind your back, try holding the end of a small towel in each hand.

2. **Take a deep breath and as you exhale, keep your arms straight and gently lift your hands toward the ceiling away from your back (see Figure 10-1b).**

   Lift your arms as high as you can while standing straight and avoiding bending forward.

3. **Hold this stretch for 30 seconds.**

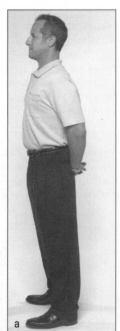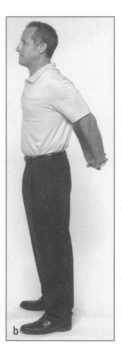

Figure 10-1:
Standing
chest
stretch.

A few do's and don't for this stretch:

- ✔ Do stand up tall with good posture.
- ✔ Do keep your knees slightly bent.
- ✔ Don't tense or lift your shoulders.

Standing abdominal stretch

After sitting for an extended period of time, the muscles in your abdomen and chest can become shortened and your back rounded. To counterbalance these effects, this stretches your chest and abdomen in the exact opposite direction, and it feels great!

To do this stretch, follow these steps:

1. **Stand with your feet shoulder-width apart and knees slightly bent.**

2. **Place your hands on the lowest part of your back, right where your buttocks meets your lower back, with your fingers pointed downward (see Figure 10-2a).**

3. **Inhale and as you exhale, squeeze your buttocks (to prevent compression in your lower back), lean back, and slightly push your hips forward (see Figure 10-2b).**

4. **Hold this stretch for 30 seconds and then come back to upright position.**

5. **Perform this exercise twice.**

Figure 10-2:
Standing abdominal stretch.

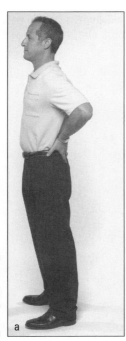
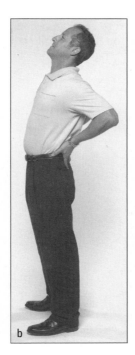

A few do's and don'ts for this stretch:

- ✔ Do squeeze your shoulder blades together as you lean back.
- ✔ Do lift your chin so your neck stays in line with the rest of your spine.
- ✔ Don't bounce or force the stretch, which puts stress on your lower back.

Standing side reach with legs crossed

After sitting for a long time, your sides get all scrunched together, so nothing can feel better than a good side reach. Feel this stretch along your rib cage and shoulders as you bring oxygen to your entire body.

To do this stretch, follow these steps:

1. **Stand tall with your arms at your sides.**

2. **Cross your left leg over your right leg, keeping both feet flat on the floor (see Figure 10-3a).**

3. **Inhale and as you exhale, lean to the left and reach your left arm toward the floor (see Figure 10-3b).**

4. **Hold the stretch for 30 seconds and then come back to starting position.**

5. **Cross your right leg over your left leg, keeping both feet on the floor and repeat the stretch leaning to the right.**

If you find it uncomfortable or awkward to cross your legs, try moving your front leg forward an inch or two. If it's still awkward, or you have trouble balancing, simply perform this stretch with your legs uncrossed and your feet together.

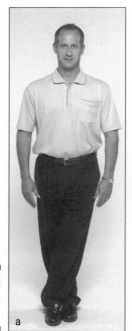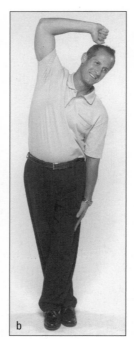

Figure 10-3:
Standing
side reach.

a

b

A few do's and don'ts for this stretch:

✔ Do keep your hips facing forward.

✔ Do keep your arms to your sides.

✔ Don't bounce or twist.

✔ Don't hold your breath, but instead breathe regularly.

Standing hamstring and calf stretch

Two areas that can get tight after sitting for a long time are the back of your thighs and your calves. This one stretch can get both areas at the same time. To perform this exercise, follow these steps:

1. **Stand tall with both feet together and your arms at your sides.**

2. **Step out with your left leg, keeping your back heel on the floor and your front toes pointing toward the ceiling.**

3. **Bend your right knee slightly and inhale.**

4. **As you exhale, hinge at your hips and tilt your pelvis back, placing both your hands just above your bent knee (see Figure 10-4).**

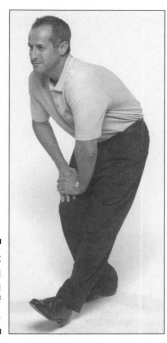

Figure 10-4:
Standing
hamstring
and calf
stretch.

5. **Hold the stretch for 30 seconds and make sure to keep your spine lengthened, your chest lifted, and your tailbone reaching toward the wall behind you.**

6. **Repeat the stretch on the other side.**

If you're not feeling the stretch in your calf, try to flex your foot more (lift your toes more toward the ceiling). If you're not feeling the stretch in your hamstrings, try tilting your pelvis back farther and lengthening your back more if you can.

A few do's and don'ts for this exercise:

✔ Do breathe slowly and rhythmically.

✔ Do keep most of your weight on your bent leg.

✔ Don't round your back or drop your chest too far toward your bent leg.

Standing hip flexor stretch

This stretch targets your hip flexors with pinpoint accuracy and, as an added bonus, can even tone your thighs and buttocks! To do this stretch, follow these steps:

1. **Start in a forward lunge position with both knees bent and your arms at your sides.**

   Make sure your feet are far enough apart so when you bend your knees your front knee doesn't jut forward past your toes.

2. **Inhale and as you exhale, squeeze your buttocks and tilt your pelvis under so your hipbones point upward and your tailbone points downward (see Figure 10-5).**

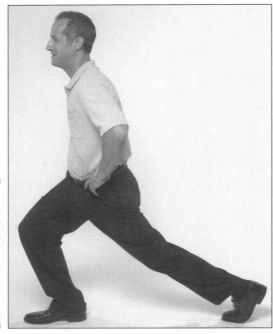

Figure 10-5: Standing hip flexor stretch — lunging forward with your pelvis tucked under.

3. **Hold the stretch for 30 seconds and then sink your hips down toward the floor to lower your body another inch or two.**

4. **Hold this lowered position for another 30 seconds, breathing comfortably and normally.**

5. **Release the stretch and bring your feet together.**

6. **Repeat the stretch on your other leg.**

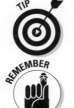

If you have trouble keeping your balance, move your back leg out to the side an inch or two. This adjustment gives you a wider base of support. Make sure your abdominals are tight and pulled in.

A few do's and don'ts for this exercise:

✔ Do keep your buttocks squeezed and your pelvis tucked under.

✔ Do keep your toes pointed forward.

✔ Do stabilize your spine by keeping your back straight and your abdominals lifted.

✔ Don't bend your knees more than 90 degrees or let your front knee jut forward. These positions place stress on your knees.

Stretches for the Professional Desk Jockey

This section gives you a few stretches to do when you can't get away from your desk. Doing these stretches several times during the day can help energize you and keep those aches and pains away.

Shoulders and neck stretch with circles

This stretch is designed to release the tension that can build up in your neck and shoulders after sitting with poor posture for too long. The shoulder circles relax your shoulders and get you sitting up tall again, while the neck stretch lengthens and relaxes the muscles in your neck. This stretch is a great if you're prone to rounded shoulders.

To do this exercise, follow these steps:

1. **Sit tall in your chair with your feet flat on the floor, your abdominals lifted, and your hands at your sides.**

2. **Slowly rotate your shoulders forward, up, back, and down as if you were drawing a circle with your shoulders (see Figure 10-6a).**

   Breathe deeply as you repeat this motion four to six times.

3. **At the end of the last repetition, hold your shoulders down and back.**

4. **Tilt your head to the left, moving your left ear toward your left shoulder.**

   Make sure you keep your right shoulder down (see Figure 10-6b).

5. **Slowly roll your head toward your chest, drawing a half circle with your chin.**

   Continue the motion until you tilt your head all the way across toward the right shoulder. Bring your head back to the upright position and relax.

6. **Repeat on the other side.**

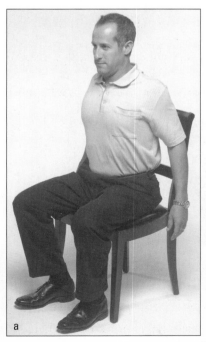 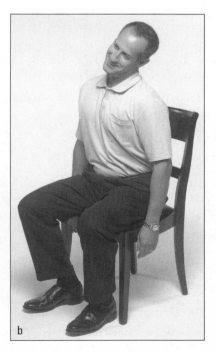

Figure 10-6: Shoulder circles and neck stretch.

a

b

A few do's and don'ts for this exercise:

- ✔ Do keep your posture tall and abdominals lifted.
- ✔ Do keep your shoulder blades down as you perform the shoulder circles.
- ✔ Don't raise one shoulder while you're performing the neck stretch. Make sure to keep both of your shoulders level at all times.

Chest stretch

If you sit for a long time, this stretch is one of the most effective ones to counteract the rounded shoulders and rounded back that can form over time (when you hover over that keyboard).

Your chest muscles tend to tighten with bad posture, which can pull your shoulders forward even more. This stretch helps stretch out those worn-out muscles and get you sitting tall again. To do this exercise, follow these steps:

1. **Sit tall with both your feet flat on the floor and your back flat against the back of your chair.**

2. **Clasp your hands together behind your head (see Figure 10-7a) and inhale.**

3. **As you exhale, gently press your elbows back, squeeze your shoulder blades together, and lift your chin and chest toward the ceiling (see Figure 10-7b).**

4. **Hold the stretch for 30 seconds and then release back to starting position.**

5. **Repeat this stretch several times each hour of sitting still or at least a few times a day.**

Figure 10-7:
Chest
stretch with
hands
behind
head.

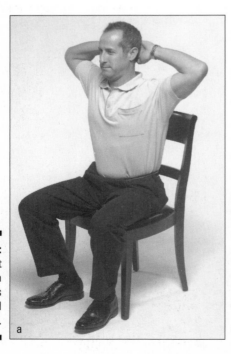
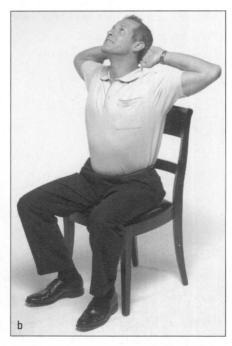

a

b

A few do's and don'ts for this exercise:

- ✔ Do breathe slowly and rhythmically.
- ✔ Do keep your chest lifted and your abdominals tight.
- ✔ Don't compress or arch your lower back.

Seated spinal rotation

Have you ever been so focused on what you're working on at your desk that you forget there is a world going on around you? Well, this stretch not only relieves tension in your hips and back, but also it's a good excuse to look up and see what's going on in the outside world.

To do this stretch follow these steps:

1. **Sit up tall in a chair with your left leg crossed over your right, your abdominals lifted, and your shoulders down (see Figure 10-8a).**

   If it's uncomfortable to cross your legs, do this stretch with both feet flat on the floor.

2. **Cross your right arm over your body so your forearm rests on your left thigh, and place your left hand on the back of the seat of your chair.**

3. **Inhale and as you exhale, twist at your waist and look back over your left shoulder.**

   Look over your shoulder as if you were trying to look behind you (see Figure 10-8b). Remember to keep your shoulders down and your gaze level.

4. **Hold the stretch for 30 seconds, gently pressing your right forearm against your left leg as you deepen the stretch.**

5. **Release the stretch and repeat on the other side by crossing your right leg over your left and twisting to the right.**

Figure 10-8: The spinal rotation that stretches your back, hips, and neck.

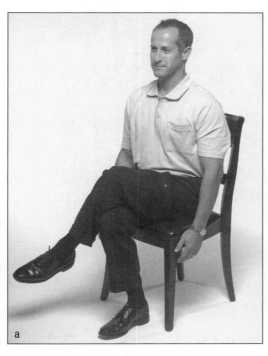
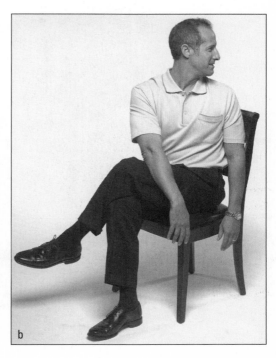

A few do's and don'ts for this exercise:

- Do sit up tall — no slouching.
- Do keep your hips facing forward.
- Don't tense up your shoulders and neck.

Seated forward bend

You should feel this stretch along the back of your legs or hamstrings. By hinging at your hips and using the weight of your upper body, you also get a good stretch in your lower back. To do this stretch, follow these steps:

1. **Sit on a chair with your feet flat on the floor and your abdominals tight (see Figure 10-9a).**

2. **Inhale and as you exhale, bend forward at the hips as far as you can comfortably stretch, letting your arms and head hang down toward the ground (see Figure 10-9b).**

3. **Hold this stretch for 30 seconds or four to five slow, deep breaths.**

4. **Slowly roll back up, stacking one vertebra on top of the other until you're sitting up tall.**

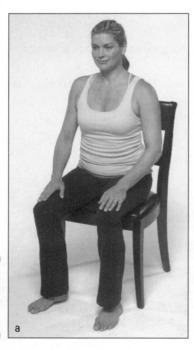
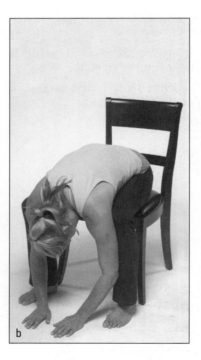

Figure 10-9:
The seated forward bend.

a

b

A few do's and don't for this stretch:

- Do feel this stretch in the back of your legs.
- Do gradually deepen the stretch with each breath.
- Don't force the stretch.

Wrist and forearm stretch

This stretch can help combat the discomfort caused by repetitive stress injuries like carpal tunnel syndrome. You should feel this stretch throughout your forearms and wrists.

To do this stretch, follow these steps:

1. **Sit up straight in your chair with the palm of one hand touching the fingers of the other hand.**

   Point your fingers upward and keep your elbows lifting toward the ceiling (see Figure 10-10).

2. **Inhale and as you exhale, gently press the heel of your hand against your fingers.**

3. **Hold this stretch for 30 seconds and repeat on the other side.**

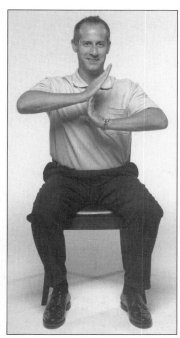

Figure 10-10: The sitting wrist and forearm stretch.

A few do's and don't for this stretch:

- ✔ Do sit up tall with good posture.
- ✔ Don't tense or lift your shoulders.
- ✔ Don't hold your breath.
- ✔ Don't let your elbows drop.

Seated ankle circles

As you get older you naturally lose range of motion in your joints, but particularly in the ankle joint. Ankle circles help increase range of motion in the joint, and they also make walking feel much more comfortable. So go ahead take your shoes off.

To do this exercise, follow these steps:

1. **Sit up tall with your feet flat on the floor.**

2. **Place your hands under your right knee and clasp them together.**

3. **Use your hands to lift your knee, lifting your foot a few inches off the floor.**

4. **Inhale and as you exhale, circle your ankle eight times inward and then eight times outward (see Figure 10-11).**

5. **Repeat this stretch on your other ankle.**

Imagine there's a pencil attached to your big toe and you're trying to draw the largest circle you can. Go slow enough so you draw a perfectly round circle.

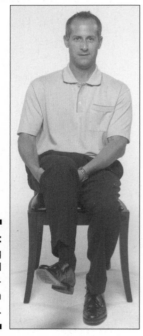

Figure 10-11:
Performing the seated ankle circles in a chair.

A few do's and don'ts for this exercise:

- ✔ Do sit up tall with your back straight.
- ✔ Do support the weight of your leg with your hands.
- ✔ Don't rush the movement.

Stress! How it affects you and your body

Excess stress can lower your immune system, make you depressed, and make you sick, but according to Pamela Peeke, MD, MPH, too much stress can also make you fat! How? Stress activates the "flight-or-fight" response, a physiological reaction designed to help your body react decisively in an emergency. When confronted with a perceived threat, your brain commands your adrenal glands to dump a large amount of the stress hormone *cortisol* into your bloodstream. One of the functions of cortisol is to quickly release energy stored in fat cells. Your muscles use the energy to help avert the emergency. The problem is that, even after the emergency is over, the level of cortisol in your bloodstream remains elevated to help encourage you to restock your stores of fat.

In addition, stressed-out women who carry weight in their abdominal area secrete significantly more cortisol than women who don't have excess fat around their waistline, according to a study from the University of California at San Francisco. And since abdominal fat tissue has up to four times the number of receptors for cortisol as does fat elsewhere in the body, the cells in this area are the most likely to store fat as a result of cortisol. Unfortunately, this excess tummy doesn't just spill over the top of your low-rise jeans; it's an indicator of increased risk for stroke and heart disease, two major killers of women over 50 years old.

What's the solution? When it comes to reducing stress, experts consistently point to regular exercise, which can also help combat cardiovascular disease. And there's nothing more effective to help you reduce the muscle tension brought on by excess stress than a good, invigorating stretch.

Chapter 11

Basic Warm-Up and Cool-Down Stretch Routines

*P*rofessional athletes, Olympic athletes, even college and high-school athletes all warm up and cool down before they practice or play. And you can take it from me that they wouldn't waste their time and effort to do so if it didn't pay off. In fact, a virtual *mountain* of research supports their experience: Warming up and cooling down enhances performance and reduces injury.

Proper stretching is one of the key components of a good warm-up and cool-down. This chapter takes these two important components and shows you how to get the best warm-up and cool-down possible for your workout.

Easing into Your Workout

So what exactly happens to your body as you increase your core temperature and prepare your muscles for exercise (warm-up!)? The following sections shed some light on why warming up is so important.

The big deal about warming up

In case you're wondering, here's what happens to your body when you warm up:

✔ Bloodflow through your muscles increases, which enhances the delivery of oxygen from your blood, and the speed of your nerve impulses increases. Both of these factors make your muscles work better.

✔ Your heart rate increases, which primes your cardiovascular system to handle the increased load from your workout.

✔ Your body and tissue temperature gently increase, which helps prevent injury by slowly increasing your body's core temperature, which allows your blood pressure to stay regulated.

> ✔ Muscular tension decreases, and your connective tissue has an enhanced ability to lengthen, which in turn enhances your performance and decreases the likelihood of injury.
>
> ✔ You slowly and gently ease into the right frame of mind for the exertion of a good workout. This mindset prevents you from getting tired out or overdoing it if you start out exercising too vigorously.

Here's what may happen if you don't warm up:

> ✔ You may pull a muscle if you start stretching out "cold" and no blood or oxygen is circulating and flowing to the area.
>
> ✔ You may become short of breath or dizzy from your heart rate increasing too quickly.
>
> ✔ You may cause injury to a joint from launching into quick movements without first loosening up the surrounding tissue.

When you try to save five minutes before you exercise and skip your warm-up, you can pull a muscle. If that happens, you can't exercise at all for two weeks while you heal (and limp around, sleep badly, and generally live with the pain). Five minutes versus two weeks — do the math. I'm no math major, but even I can see that warming up before you work out makes more sense than not doing so.

Making stretching a part of your warm-up

Like a good play or movie, a good warm-up has three acts or phases. These three phases are important because, first, they mimic the movements you'll be doing in a slower, less vigorous fashion to help prevent injury. Second, the dynamic moves allow you to increase your range of motion. And finally, the static stretching phase helps you increase muscle length, which results in increased flexibility.

In this case, the three acts are as follows:

1. **The rehearsal phase:** In this phase, you should perform moves that mimic what your workout will be. For example:

   • If you're going jogging, start with a very light trot or walk.

   • If you're going to play tennis, spend a few minutes volleying the ball back and forth.

   • If you're taking an aerobics class, spend a few minutes doing light choreography.

2. **The dynamic stretching phase:** This phase refers to general, full-body moves that aren't directly related to your intended activity. Such moves should be large range-of-motion moves, traveling through all three planes of motion. They should be dynamic in nature, fluid, and rhythmic.

3. **The multijoint static stretching phase:** After a few minutes of mimicking your workout, and then going through some integrated, dynamic stretches, your body will be warm enough to perform a few multimuscle static stretches to introduce length to the muscles and mobility to the joints.

Never start your warm-up with static stretches. Always take a few minutes to perform the rehearsal moves and the general dynamic stretches before moving into the final static phase.

Practicing your balancing act

For what it's worth, my personal preference is to include one or two balance exercises at the end of your warm-up and cool-down (I include one such exercise at the end of the warm-up routine). The warm-up can create internal heat and mental focus. The cool-down can be a bridge between the workout and slow stretches. Balance is like everything else — either use it or lose it!

Keep in mind that the goal of stretching in the warm-up isn't specifically to increase flexibility — it's to generally warm up the body and introduce the range of motion that the upcoming workout requires of your muscles. Therefore, don't hold the stretches in the warm-up for as long as you do in the cool-down, and never leave your comfort zone.

A Great Routine to Warm Your Body

The moves you perform in the rehearsal phase of your warm-up are up to you and should closely mimic the moves you make in your sport or workout. After you complete the rehearsal phase of your warm-up, move into dynamic stretches and then static stretches. This section gives you some of my favorite dynamic and static stretches for warm-up.

Dynamic stretches for the warm-up

The purpose of dynamic stretches is to warm your muscles and loosen your joints. This section provides you with three functional, dynamic stretches to do before any workout. They add on to the work you accomplish in the rehearsal phase of your warm-up by continuing to warm up your entire body, introducing range of motion to your joints, and lengthening your muscles.

Alternating knee lifts

Alternating knee lifts are meant to not only warm up your entire body but also to give you a great dynamic stretch in your hips, buttocks, thighs, and lower back.

To do this stretch, follow these steps:

1. **Stand tall with your feet together and your hands to your side.**

2. **Inhale and as you exhale, lift your left knee toward your chest (see Figure 11-1a).**

3. **Grab underneath your knee with both hands to lift your leg a little higher.**

   Actively use your hands to lift your knee as close to your chest as possible. Lifting your knee a tiny bit higher stretches your buttocks and hamstrings a lot more.

4. **Lower your leg down to starting position and repeat the exercise on your other leg (see Figure 11-1b).**

5. **Repeat the stretch for 16 to 20 repetitions.**

For a simple variation, lift your knees to the side rather than forward. As you become more advanced, try to raise up on the toes of the foot on the floor.

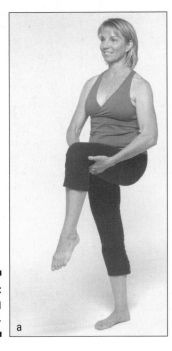 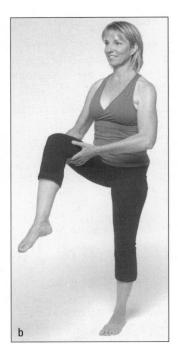

Figure 11-1:
Alternating
knee lifts.

a   b

A few do's and don'ts for this stretch:

- ✔ Do stand up tall and bring your knee to your chest, not your chest to your knee.
- ✔ Do exhale every time you lift your knee.
- ✔ Do keep your chest lifted and shoulder blades down.
- ✔ Don't grab the top of your kneecap.
- ✔ Don't tilt your pelvis under.
- ✔ Don't yank or forcefully pull on your knee — the movement should be smooth.

Torso twists

This stretch warms up your whole body, as well as stretches your abs, back, and shoulders. It also prepares your body for any twisting or reaching that many sports and activities require.

To do this stretch, follow these steps:

1. **Stand tall with your feet apart, your abs and chest lifted, your shoulders back and down, and your hands clasped together at chest level (see Figure 11-2a).**

2. **Inhale and as you exhale, bend your knees and pivot on your left big toe, turning your hips and shoulders to the right (see Figure 11-2b).**

   Keep your feet wide and your knees bent. This stance keeps your center of gravity low and makes keeping your upper body relaxed easier.

3. **Repeat on the left side (see Figure 11-2c).**

4. **Repeat the stretch for 16 to 20 repetitions, keeping your arms and shoulders relaxed so that the momentum of hips moves your elbows behind you.**

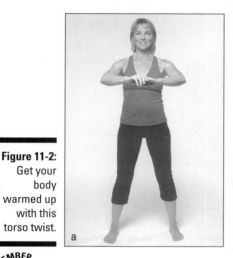
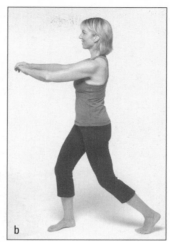
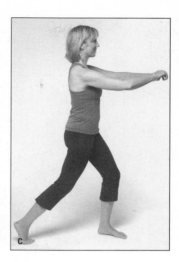

Figure 11-2: Get your body warmed up with this torso twist.

A few do's and don'ts for this stretch:

- ✔ Do keep your knees bent at all times.
- ✔ Do keep your abdominals lifted.
- ✔ Don't force or jerk the movement, because the movement should flow from side to side.
- ✔ Don't lock your knees or keep your hips facing the front.

The chop

The chop, which is so named because it sort of looks like the move a person makes when chopping wood, is the king of all functional stretches because it stretches your buttocks, back, abs, and chest all at the same time. This stretch also prepares your body for any twisting, reaching, or bending you may be doing in your workout.

To do this stretch, follow these steps:

1. **Stand up tall with your feet hip-width apart and your arms at your sides.**

2. **Bend your knees and pivot on your left big toe as you lift your left heel.**

   Your right foot remains on the ground and faces forward (see Figure 11-3a).

3. **Twist your hips to the right and reach both of your arms down and behind you.**

4. **Hold the position for one long, deep breath.**

5. **Come back to center and continue to turn your hips as you reach both arms overhead to the left (see Figure 11-3b).**

6. **Hold this position for one long, deep breath.**

   You should feel the stretch in your right hip flexor, obliques, and chest.

7. **Repeat the stretch from right to left for six to eight repetitions, and as you get stronger, work your way up to two sets of eight repetitions.**

To protect your back and spine, your hips should move with you and not remain forward throughout the moves.

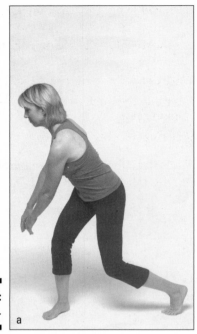
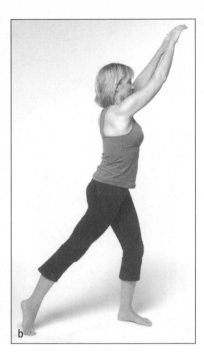

Figure 11-3: The chop.

a

b

A few do's and don'ts for this stretch:

✔ Do inhale as you reach up, and exhale as you bring your arm back down.

✔ Do lengthen your spine throughout the movement.

✔ Do hold your abdominals tight to protect your back.

✔ Don't arch or compress your lower back.

✔ Don't let your knees bow in or collapse inward.

✔ Don't swing or create too much momentum; keep the movement fluid and under control.

Static stretches for the warm-up

The next three exercises are static stretches to introduce the range of motion that your muscles and joints are doing in the workout.

Remember, the stretches in a warm-up are to just introduce range of motion, not to increase flexibility. Therefore, you won't hold these stretches for as long as you would after your workout.

Standing calf and hip flexor stretch

Stretching the calf and the hip flexor together is valuable because they affect each other. If your calf is tight, it may limit the movement in your hip flexor. If your hip flexor is tight, then it may limit your range of motion in your calf.

To do this stretch, follow these steps:

1. **Stand tall with your left foot back far enough to still keep your heel on the ground (see Figure 11-4a).**

2. **Bend your right knee and reach your left arm overhead as you press your hip forward (see Figure 11-4b).**

3. **Squeeze your buttocks to feel the stretch a little deeper in your hip flexor and calf.**

   As you stretch your arm overhead and press your hip forward, you should feel as if your spine is lengthening, not shortening or compressing.

4. **Hold the stretch for 30 seconds and then repeat on your other leg.**

To make this stretch more dynamic, alternate it with the hamstring/back stretch in Figure 11-5 later in the chapter.

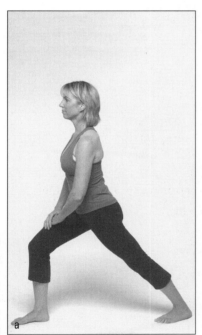 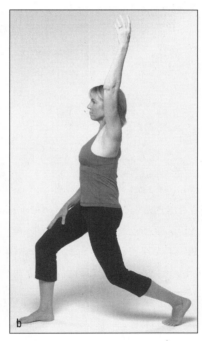

Figure 11-4: The standing calf and hip flexor stretch.

A few do's and don'ts for this stretch:

- Do reach up and back, not just back.
- Do work on getting your heel to stay on the ground.
- Don't arch your back.
- Don't relax your abdominal muscles — keep your bellybutton toward your spine.

Hamstring and back stretch

You should feel this stretch throughout your entire backside — heel, calf, hamstring, lower back, and lats. Try not to tighten your shoulders and round your back during this stretch.

Stay in your comfort zone during this stretch. Remember that you're introducing range of motion, not trying to increase your overall flexibility.

To do this stretch, follow these steps:

1. **Stand with your feet in a wide stance about hip-width apart.**

2. **Extend your left leg so your heel on your right leg remains on the floor and your toes on the left leg are lifted toward the ceiling.**

3. **Bend your right knee as you slowly press your hips back (see Figure 11-5a).**

4. **Reach your right hand toward your left toes or the outside of your left leg (see Figure 11-5b.**

5. **Hold the stretch for 30 seconds and then repeat on the other side.**

To make this stretch more dynamic, alternate it with the standing calf and hip flexor stretch in Figure 11-4.

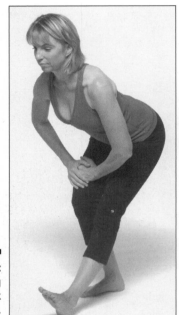 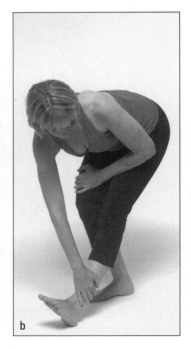

Figure 11-5: Hamstring and back stretch.

a   b

A few do's and don'ts for this stretch:

✔ Do tilt your pelvis back.

✔ Do try to keep your back flat.

✔ Do keep your foot flexed and your toes pointed up.

✔ Don't bounce or force the stretch.

✔ Don't tighten up your shoulders or round your back.

Standing groin and inner thigh stretch

This stretch is for the muscles that run along your inner thigh and also the muscles in your torso that rotate your spine. This stretch also builds strength in your thighs and creates heat in your body so your muscles are nice and warm for a productive, pain-free workout.

To do this stretch, follow these steps:

1. **Stand with your feet in a wide stance with your toes pointing out.**

2. **Bend your knees and slowly lean forward until your elbows can rest just inside your knees (see Figure 11-6a).**

3. **Gently press your right elbow against the inside of your right knee as you lower your right shoulder and rotate your spine to the left, looking over your left shoulder (see Figure 11-6b).**

   Turning your head stretches your neck muscles at the same time other muscles are stretching during this exercise.

4. **Lower your hips another inch and tilt your pelvis back.**

   Lowering your hips deepens the stretch in your groin. Think of reaching your tailbone to the ceiling as you tilt your pelvis back.

5. **Hold the stretch for 30 seconds and then repeat the stretch on the other side.**

To make this stretch more dynamic, alternate from side to side several times without holding the stretch.

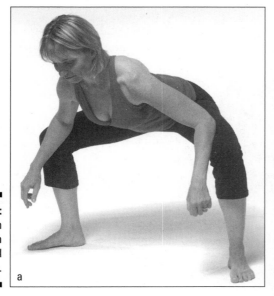
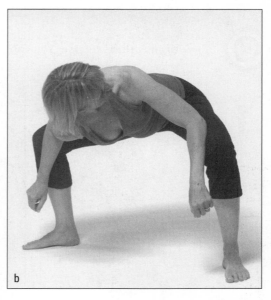

Figure 11-6: Inner thigh stretch with spinal rotation.

a

b

A few do's and don'ts for this stretch:

- ✔ Do breathe as you hold the stretch.
- ✔ Do press the knee away with your elbow.
- ✔ Do tilt your pelvis back.
- ✔ Don't hold your breath.
- ✔ Don't bounce or force the stretch.

Standing balance with a twist

Adding a little balance work to your warm-up can raise your internal temperature and improve your balance. Try this exercise *before* your next workout.

To do this stretch, follow these steps:

1. **Stand tall with your feet together and your arms at your side.**

2. **Shift your weight to your right leg only.**

3. **Bend your left knee slightly and lift your foot off the floor so all your weight is on your right leg (see Figure 11-7a).**

4. **Inhale and as you exhale, raise your elbows and cross your arms in front of your chest.**

5. **Twist to your left, hold for a few seconds, and return back to front position (see Figure 11-7b).**

   Don't attempt the twist until you're stable on one foot. If you're wobbly, use a chair or barre to help with your stability. Don't be afraid of a little wobble; it's how you test your limits and improve your balance.

6. **Repeat this exercise three more times and then repeat four repetitions on the other side.**

To make this exercise more challenging, try standing on a *bosu* — a balance board — while performing this exercise. You can find a bosu at pretty much any sporting goods store.

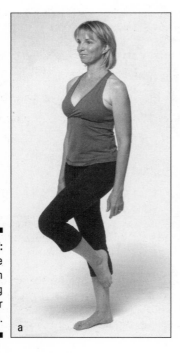
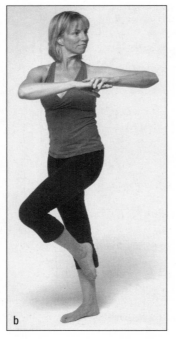

Figure 11-7: An exercise to work on improving your balance.

A few do's and don'ts for this stretch:

- ✔ Do exhale every time you twist.

- ✔ Do keep your hips level with each other. If one hip is higher than the other, holding your balance becomes difficult.

- ✔ Do hold your abdominals tight and your shoulder blades down.

- ✔ Don't lift your foot too high — only a couple of inches off the floor.

Moving Out of Your Exercise Session: Why and How to Cool Down

A *cool-down* refers to a group of moves or stretches performed after exercise and before rest. This time is perfect to work on increasing flexibility because the temperature of your muscles and connective tissue is highest, which means that these structures are now at their most flexible.

The type of stretches most appropriate for the cool-down is static stretches. Static stretches help relax your muscles by lengthening them. They can also aid in reducing after-exercise muscle soreness by helping to work lactic acid out of your muscles. In addition, a nice quiet period of gentle movement and rest can be the perfect ending to a great workout.

Why cool down? During a strenuous workout, your body goes through a number of stressful processes. Here are a few reasons why a good cool-down is so important:

- ✔ To promote recovery and return the body to its state before exercise.

- ✔ To prevent damage to the muscle fibers, tendons, and ligaments.

- ✔ To prevent the build up of lactic acid and other waste products within your body.

- ✔ To reduce soreness by keeping the blood from "pooling" or staying in the muscle. Instead, the blood gets pushed back to the heart.

Basic Cool-Down Routine

This routine is designed to stretch your body from head to toe after your workout. You can do this cool-down at the gym or at home, and most of the stretches are done on the floor, so grab a mat or find a carpeted space to make sure that you're comfortable.

I suggest that you remove your shoes to make yourself more comfortable before beginning this cool-down. Drinking water also keeps you from getting dehydrated and replaces the lost fluids from your sweat during your workout. Aim for 8 to 16 ounces of water to help you recover and reduce muscle soreness. Also have a towel or strap handy for some of these stretches.

Seated side reach

This cool-down routine focuses on your waist and stretches out the obliques — the muscles that run down the side of your body. To do this stretch, follow these steps:

1. **Sit on the floor with your legs crossed in front of you.**

2. **Reach your left arm directly overhead, using the muscles in your upper back to keep your shoulder blade down and chest lifted.**

   This position keeps space between your shoulder and ear (see Figure 11-8a).

3. **Inhale and as you exhale, bend at the waist to the right and reach with your left arm overhead, keeping your hip anchored to the floor.**

   Rest your right hand on the floor for extra support (see Figure 11-8b). Think of both sides of your waist lifting and lengthening up and over.

4. **Hold this stretch for 30 seconds or four to five slow, deep breaths.**

   Try to deepen the stretch with every breath.

5. **Repeat this stretch on your other side.**

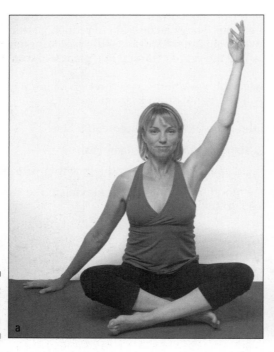 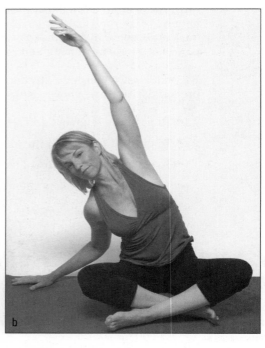

Figure 11-8: Seated side reach.

A few do's and don'ts for this stretch:

✔ Do keep your hip anchored to the floor.

✔ Do breathe and slowly deepen the stretch.

✔ Do keep your chest and shoulders facing forward.

✔ Don't bend forward or arch your back.

✔ Don't hold your breath.

Seated back and neck stretch

The best part about this stretch is that you'll feel it not only in your hips but also along your entire back and up through your neck. To do this stretch, follow these steps:

1. **Sit on the floor with your legs crossed in front of you and your hands on the floor in front of your legs (see Figure 11-9a).**

   If you feel pain in your hips or knees while sitting on the floor, raise your hips off the floor by sitting on a pillow, folded blanket, step, or bosu.

2. **Inhale and as you exhale bend forward at your hips and use your hands and arms for support.**

   With each breath, deepen the stretch by gently reaching forward with your arms (see Figure 11-9b).

3. **Hold the position in Step 2 and drop your chin toward your chest.**

4. **Shake your head "no" to release muscle tension in your neck.**

5. **Tilt your head to the right and hold the stretch for a few deep breaths.**

6. **Tilt your head to the left and hold the stretch for a few deep breaths.**

7. **Release the neck stretch and slowly sit up.**

Don't always do this stretch with the same leg crossed on top; sometimes have your right leg on top and sometimes have your left leg crossed on top. This variation keeps the stretch balanced for both hips.

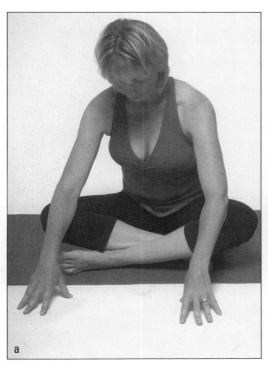
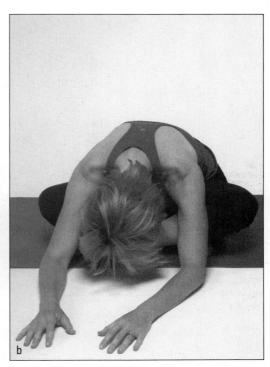

Figure 11-9: Seated cross-legged back and neck stretch.

a

b

A few do's and don'ts for this stretch:

- ✔ Do initiate the movement from your hips, not from your upper back.
- ✔ Do keep your chin down as you tilt to the side.
- ✔ Don't tense or tighten your shoulders or back.

Butterfly stretch

This stretch is for the muscles that run along your inner thigh and groin. To do this stretch, follow these steps:

1. **Sit on the floor with your back straight, your abdominals in, and the soles of your feet touching each other.**

   It's important to keep your back straight during this stretch because rounding your back places undue pressure on your lower back and spine. Sit up tall and think of your chest lifting forward as you tilt your pelvis back.

2. **Place your hands on your ankles and bring your feet as close to your groin as you can (see Figure 11-10a).**

3. **Inhale and as you exhale, gently press down on the inside of your knees with your elbows (see Figure 11-10b).**

4. **Hold this stretch for 30 seconds or four to five slow, deep breaths.**

   With each breath, try to get your knees closer to the floor.

Figure 11-10:
The butterfly stretch works your inner thigh and groin area.

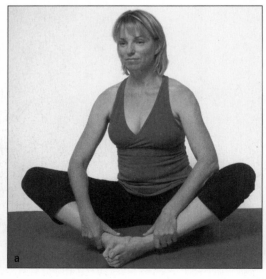
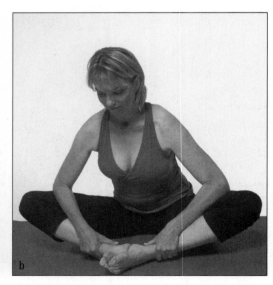
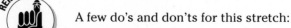

A few do's and don'ts for this stretch:

- ✔ Do breathe as you hold the stretch.
- ✔ Do lengthen your spine as you lean forward from the hips.

✔ Do keep your neck in line with the rest of your spine. You should be looking at the floor in front of you, not at your feet.

✔ Don't round your back or tighten your shoulders.

✔ Don't bounce your knees toward the floor — be patient and hold the stretch.

Seated hamstring stretch

Most people find it more comfortable and effective to perform this stretch with the aid of a towel or strap. To do this stretch, follow these steps:

1. **Sit on the floor with your right leg straight out in front of you and your left leg bent at a comfortable angle (see Figure 11-11a).**

2. **As you exhale, hinge forward at the hip, keeping your leg straight and your foot flexed (see Figure 11-11b).**

   Pay close attention to the position of your pelvis. Your tailbone should be reaching back as you hinge forward at the hips. Don't get discouraged if your chest is nowhere near your leg. As long as you're feeling a good deep stretch in the back of your thigh, you're doing great!

3. **Breathe deeply and hold the stretch for 30 seconds.**

   Deepen the stretch with each breath by tilting your pelvis back, lifting your chest, and flexing your foot forward.

4. **Repeat the same stretch on your left leg.**

Figure 11-11: The seated hamstring stretch.

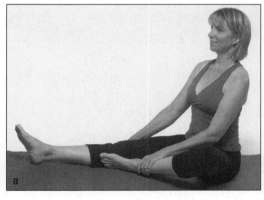 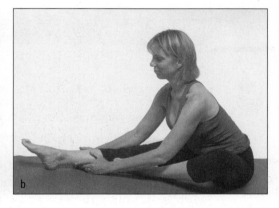

A few do's and don'ts for this stretch:

✔ Do gently pull your foot toward your body with the towel or strap.

✔ Do keep your knee straight, and try to keep the back of your knee on the floor.

✔ Do keep your back straight, not rounded or tensed in your shoulders.

✔ Don't force the stretch or pull too hard on the towel.

✔ Don't look down at your knees; look at the floor in front of your toes.

Seated twist with one leg extended

This stretch gives you a rotational stretch for your core and a stretch in your buttocks at the same time. To do this stretch, follow these steps:

1. **Sit on the floor with your right leg straight in front of you, your left foot crossed over your right thigh, and your hands on the floor behind you (see Figure 11-12a).**

2. **As you inhale, bring your right knee toward your chest and sit up very straight, lengthening your spine (see Figure 11-12b).**

3. **As you exhale, look over your left shoulder, rotate your spine, and tilt your pelvis back.**

   Pay close attention to the position of your pelvis. If you avoid tucking your pelvis under, and you really think about your tailbone reaching for the wall behind you, then you stretch your abs and back, but you also feel a stretch deep in your buttocks.

4. **Hold the stretch for 30 seconds, deepening the stretch with every breath.**

5. **Switch sides and repeat the same stretch on your other leg.**

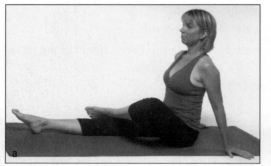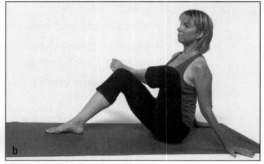

Figure 11-12: Seated twist with an added buttocks stretch.

A few do's and don'ts for this stretch:

- ✓ Do bring your knee close to your chest before you twist.
- ✓ Do look over your shoulder to lengthen your neck muscles, too.
- ✓ Do lengthen your spine before you rotate.
- ✓ Don't tuck your pelvis under or round your back.

Seated straddle stretch

This stretch integrates many muscle groups — inner thigh, back, hamstrings — into one stretch. To do this stretch, follow these steps:

1. **Sit on the floor with your legs straight, your feet as far apart as possible, and your hands behind your hips; sit up very tall (see Figure 11-13a).**

   Keeping your hands behind your hips helps you keep your spine lifted and straight. This position allows you to stretch your back, inner thighs, and hamstrings without creating tension in your shoulders and upper back.

2. **Move your hips forward an inch or two until you feel the stretch along both inner thighs.**

3. **Inhale and as you exhale lean slightly forward, tilting your pelvis back (see Figure 11-13b).**

   Your hands are behind your hips in this step, but if you want to add a variation and you're flexible enough to bring your hands in front of you without rounding your back, you can deepen the stretch by reaching forward as far as you can.

4. **Hold the stretch for 30 seconds or four to five slow, deep breaths.**

Your goal isn't to get your chest to the floor; it's to feel a stretch in your inner thighs without your pelvis tucking under or your back rounding or your knees rolling inward. Even though this stretch is common, it can still be difficult because of all the muscles involved.

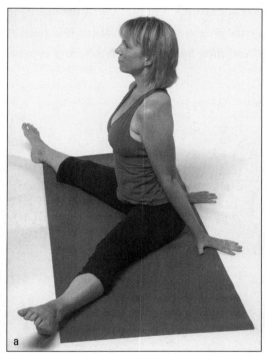
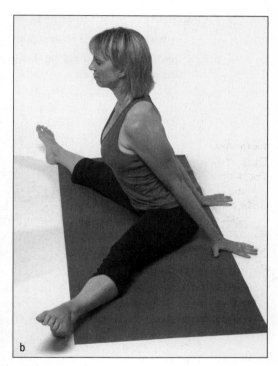

Figure 11-13:
The seated straddle stretch.

a

b

A few do's and don'ts for this stretch:

✔ Do keep your knees and toes facing upward toward the ceiling.

✔ Do tilt your pelvis back as you lift your chest.

✔ Do breathe deeply through the entire stretch.

✔ Do progress slowly through this stretch, spending 15 seconds or so in the comfort zone.

✔ Don't place your hands in front of you unless you can keep them there without rounding your spine or tucking your pelvis under.

✔ Don't bounce this stretch.

Side lying quad stretch

This quad stretch is one of the easiest stretches to get into and maintain proper form. You should feel this stretch in your back, obliques, neck, and chest all at the same time.

To do this stretch, follow these steps:

1. **Lie on your right side with your knees bent close to your chest, and let your head rest on your right arm (see Figure 11-14a).**

2. **Grab the top of your left foot and gently move your ankle back toward your buttocks (see Figure 11-14b).**

   Don't force your heel toward your buttocks. That movement can put pressure on your knee joint.

3. **Squeeze your buttocks to increase the stretch, but don't let your hips roll back.**

   Always keep your hips stacked on top of each other and focus on bringing the knee back.

4. **Hold the stretch for 30 seconds, and then lie on your left side and repeat the stretch on your other leg.**

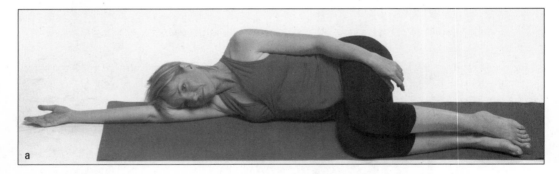

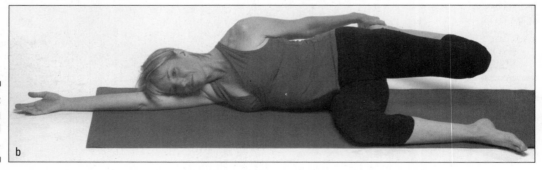

Figure 11-14:
Side lying
quad
stretch.

A few do's and don'ts for this stretch:

✔ Do breathe as you hold the stretch.

✔ Do squeeze your buttocks to deepen the stretch.

✔ Don't jam your heel toward your buttocks.

- ✔ Do keep your bottom knee bent for balance.
- ✔ Don't lift the knee — instead try to keep your inner thighs touching.

Back extension and abdominal stretch

This stretch is specifically for the abdominals, but it's also great for the back muscles. The back extension and abdominal stretch increases mobility in your spine and decreases a rounded back.

To do this stretch, follow these steps:

1. **Lie on your belly, supporting your upper body with your elbows directly under your shoulders.**

2. **Lift up out of your shoulders so you aren't sinking into your shoulder blades.**

3. **Inhale and as you exhale, lengthen your spine and lift your chest as if you were going to move forward (see Figure 11-15).**

   Imagine you're trying to move forward, but your elbows and hips are glued to the floor. And visualize the space between each vertebra as increasing, lengthening your spine. You should feel this stretch in your abdominals.

4. **Hold the stretch for 30 seconds or four to five slow, deep breaths.**

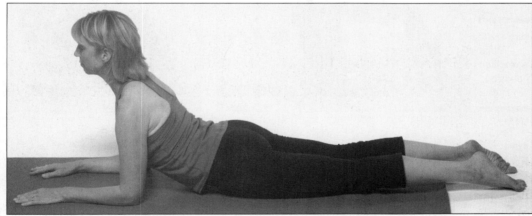

Figure 11-15:
Back extension and abdominal stretch.

A few do's and don'ts for this stretch:

- ✔ Do keep your neck long and in line with the rest of your spine.
- ✔ Do keep your shoulder blades down.
- ✔ Do pull your belly toward your spine.
- ✔ Don't compress your lower back.
- ✔ Don't think of lifting your chest toward the ceiling; think of your chest pressing up toward the ceiling.

Wrist stretch on all fours

This stretch is my favorite for the wrist and forearm areas; if you have carpal tunnel syndrome, though, you should skip this one. To do this stretch, follow these steps:

1. **Kneel on all fours with most of your weight on your knees.**

2. **Place your left hand palm down, fingers facing back toward your knee (see figure 11-16a).**

3. **Inhale and as you exhale, gently shift your body weight toward your shoulders.**

4. **Hold the stretch for 30 seconds or four to five slow, deep breaths.**

   Feel the stretch in the palm of your right hand and forearm.

5. **Release the stretch and place the back of your hand on the floor with your fingers toward your knee (see Figure 11-16b).**

6. **Hold this stretch for 30 seconds or four to five slow, deep breaths.**

7. **Repeat these two stretches on your other wrist.**

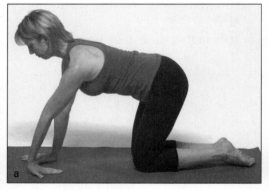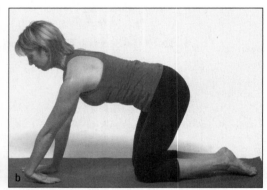

Figure 11-16:
Wrist stretch on hands and knees.

A few do's and don'ts for this stretch:

✔ Do keep your shoulder blades down and your body weight shifted toward your heels.

✔ Don't put all your weight on the wrist being stretched.

✔ Don't bounce during the stretch.

Hip flexor stretch on one knee

The benefit of this stretch is that it can target your hip flexor — a very difficult muscle to isolate but one that's important to stretch because it's responsible for how you walk and all lower body movement.

If this kneeling stretch is uncomfortable on your knees, try placing a folded towel or pillow under your knee for cushion.

To do this stretch, follow these steps:

1. **Kneel on one knee, place your other foot flat on the floor in front of you with your knee bent, and make sure you maintain good posture with your upper body.**

   Make sure that the back foot and leg aren't turned in. You'll feel the stretch a little more in your hip flexor if your foot is directly behind your hip.

2. **Inhale and as you exhale, squeeze your buttocks and tilt your pelvis under (see Figure 11-17).**

   Feel the front part of your hip lengthen. If you don't feel the stretch, you may have to squeeze your buttocks and tuck your pelvis a little more.

3. **Hold the stretch for 30 seconds or four to five slow, deep breaths.**

4. **Repeat on the other side.**

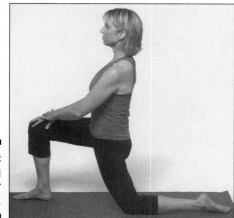

Figure 11-17: Kneeling hip flexor stretch.

A few do's and don'ts for this stretch:

- ✔ Do breathe throughout the stretch.
- ✔ Do keep your chest lifted and shoulders back.
- ✔ Do keep your shoulders directly over your hips — you want to lengthen the front of your hip, not shorten it.
- ✔ Don't hinge forward at your hip.
- ✔ Don't arch your back; just focus on squeezing your buttocks and tucking your pelvis under.

Chapter 12

My Favorite Stretches for Specific Sports

*T*hink for a moment about an unbelievable catch in baseball or football or an amazing return in tennis. All these feats require a combination of power, agility, and coordination. And yet if athletes didn't have the flexibility to reach and stretch their bodies that last little bit, they never would've been able to make the play. And what's more, if they weren't extremely limber, reaching to the utmost limit would most likely cause an injury.

Whether you're a professional athlete or an aging weekend warrior, anyone who engages in a sport can benefit from stretching — the key to not only enhanced performance but also to long-term, injury-free fun.

I chose the stretches in this chapter to address the specific movements required in a given sport, but it's not enough to only stretch one area of the body. Along with the two stretches I show you for each sport, your overall flexibility program should include stretches for your neck, shoulders, back, buttocks, hip flexors, thighs, and lower legs. Check out Chapter 8 and Chapter 11 for examples of total body stretch routines you can do regularly.

Guidelines You Don't Want to Skip

No matter what sport you engage in, you want to improve your athletic performance and decrease your risk of injury. So check out the following list for some basic flexibility training guidelines:

- ✔ **Warm up.** Make sure you warm up *before* you start to exercise. You need just about 10 to 15 minutes of dynamic stretching that mimics what you'll later be doing full speed. Check out Chapter 11 for some examples of dynamic warm-up stretches.

- ✔ **Drink fluids.** Your muscles and joints need fluid to stay flexible and lubricated. So here are the guidelines:

  - If you exercise for less than an hour, water is more than adequate.

  - However, if you exercise more than an hour, a sports drink improves endurance, reaction time, and concentration because carbohydrates are being used by both the brain and muscle during prolonged exercise.

- ✔ **Focus on a particular area.** Each sport has specific requirements: A runner needs a flexible lower body; racquet sports require flexibility in the upper body; and in contact sports, you need a strong flexible core. To enhance performance and help prevent injury, focus on the area you use the most.

- ✔ **Don't forget the rest of your body.** If you're serious about improving your game through stretching, you'll have to engage in a flexibility program that stretches your entire body two or three days a week. Like everything else in life, you get out of it what you put into it.

- ✔ **Cool down.** Never forget to cool down after a workout because it allows the blood and oxygen to return to your heart and muscles instead of "pooling" or staying in your extremities. After your breathing returns to normal and your heart rate is under 100 beats per minute, your body has cooled down sufficiently.

Running and Hiking

When you go for a run or a hike, you use the powerhouse muscles or large muscle groups in the lower half. These muscles need stretching so they can support all the dynamic movements your body demands. The following two stretches focus on the large, powerful muscles in the lower body to make sure that your body is as balanced as possible.

Gluteal stretch

One of the main functions of the gluteal muscles of the buttocks is to help fully extend the hip joint, which is a crucial part of the running motion. This exercise helps ensure that you get full range of motion in your buttocks muscles, and therefore your hips, which results in a long, graceful, fluid, powerful running stride.

To do this stretch, follow these steps:

1. **Get on the floor on your hands and knees.**

2. **Bring your left knee forward as far as you can, and rest your knee, shin and foot on the floor.**

3. **Inhale and as you exhale, lower your left buttock to the ground, extending your right leg behind you and resting the front of your right thigh, kneecap, shin, and foot on the floor (see Figure 12-1).**

4. **Gently push your right hip toward the floor and hold the stretch for 30 seconds.**

   To intensify this stretch, try moving your front foot farther away from your hip.

5. **Repeat this stretch on your other leg.**

A few do's and don'ts for this stretch:

- ✔ Do keep your hips facing front.

- ✔ Do support the weight of your upper body on your hands.

- ✔ Do lean forward, but don't arch your back.

- ✔ Don't continue holding the stretch if you feel pain in your front knee.

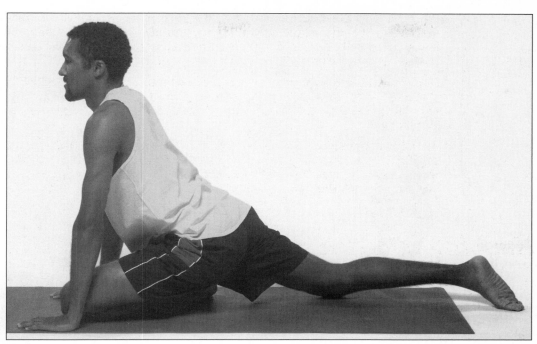

Figure 12-1:
The gluteal
stretch.

Calf stretch

To make sure you fully address both of the major calf muscles — the gastrocnemius and the soleus — perform this stretch in both positions: with your leg straight and with your knee slightly bent.

Always begin the calf stretch in the comfort zone for the first 10 to 15 seconds of the stretch. This period allows your body to get comfortable with the stretch and gives your muscles a chance to relax and let go before you try to deepen the stretch. For this reason, I recommend performing this stretch in the warm-up period of your workout.

To do this stretch, follow these steps:

1. **Stand with one foot flat on the landing of a step or the top of a curb.**

2. **Place only the ball of your other foot on the edge of the step, slightly behind the first foot (see Figure 12-2).**

3. **Slowly let your heel lower below the edge of the step until you feel tension in your calf.**

4. **Hold the stretch for 15 seconds as you breathe deeply.**

5. **Inhale and as you exhale, bend your back knee slightly, keeping your heel reaching toward the floor.**

   This stretch mimics the ankle and calf position during running. Using a step helps increase the range of motion in your ankle joint. You may need to hold on to a staircase railing or a sturdy surface nearby to help you keep your balance.

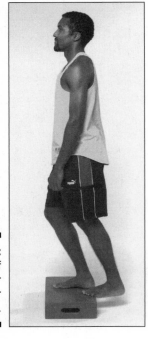

Figure 12-2:
The calf
stretch for
runners or
hikers.

6. **Hold the stretch for another 15 to 20 seconds, keeping your shoulders down and chest lifted.**

   If you lean forward slightly during the stretch, the stretch will deepen.

7. **Repeat this stretch on the other leg.**

A few do's and don'ts for this stretch:

   ✔ Do progress through the stretch gradually.

   ✔ Do lean forward so you don't lose your balance.

   ✔ Don't bounce or force the stretch.

Racquet Sports

If you play racquet sports, you may notice that you generally use one side of your body — or the dominant arm — more than the other, thus creating an imbalance, or asymmetry, between your two sides. When training for racquet sports, remember to always strengthen and stretch both sides equally because an imbalance can lead to injury.

Wrist and forearm stretch

This stretch can help prevent tennis elbow — a painful inflammation of the tissue surrounding the elbow, caused by strain from playing tennis and other sports and from overuse of the lower arm muscles — because it lengthens the forearm muscles. You feel this stretch not only in your forearms but also in your wrists and hands.

To do this stretch, follow these steps:

1. **Stand tall with your back straight and your feet a comfortable distance apart.**

2. **Relax your shoulders and lift your abdominals.**

3. **Inhale and extend your right arm forward about shoulder height, palm up.**

4. **As you exhale, grab the fingers of your right hand with your left hand and gently pull your fingers back toward your body (see Figure 12-3a).**

5. **Hold this stretch for 10 to 15 seconds, breathing deeply throughout the stretch.**

6. **Release the stretch and rotate your palm face down.**

7. **Inhale and use your left hand to gently pull the tips of your right fingers back toward your body (see Figure 12-3b).**

8. **Hold this stretch for 10 to 15 seconds, breathing deeply throughout the stretch.**

9. **Repeat the stretch on the left arm.**

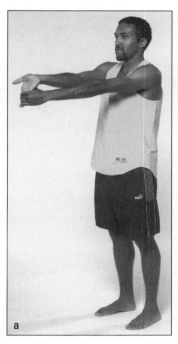
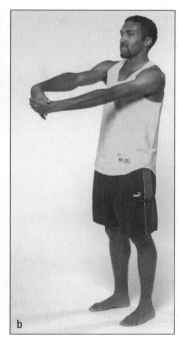

Figure 12-3:
The wrist and forearm stretch helps prevent tennis elbow.

A few do's and don'ts for this stretch:

✔ Do sit up tall with your feet flat on the floor.

✔ Do keep your arms extended as you stretch the wrist.

✔ Do breathe through the stretch.

✔ Don't hold the stretch if you feel pain in your wrist joint.

Kneeling chest stretch

The following stretch increases shoulder range of motion by lengthening and stretching the largest of your chest muscles — the pectoralis major. Perform the following steps for the kneeling chest stretch:

1. **Kneel on a carpeted floor or mat with your forearms crossed and resting on the seat of a sturdy chair (see Figure 12-4a).**

2. **Breathe in and as you exhale let your head and chest sink below the chair (see Figure 12-4b).**

3. **Hold the stretch for 30 seconds.**

   You should feel the stretch in your upper chest and use deep breathing to help sink gradually deeper into the stretch.

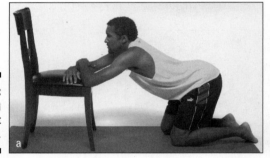
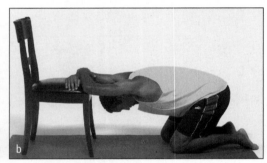

Figure 12-4: Kneeling chest stretch.

A few do's and don'ts for this stretch:

- ✔ Do start the stretch in the comfort zone and gradually progress into a deep stretch.
- ✔ Do maintain the natural curve of you spine, avoiding arching or rounding your back.
- ✔ Do lift your bellybutton toward your spine.
- ✔ Don't allow your pelvis to tilt back or tuck under.
- ✔ Don't do this stretch if it causes shoulder pain.

Basketball

Basketball is truly a total-body sport that requires some very specific movements to shoot the ball and move with maximum mobility. The stretches in this section help increase your overhead reach to snag rebounds and improve the range of motion in your triceps to help you drain those jump shots.

Step back with overhead reach

This stretch is for the muscles that run along the front of your torso. You should feel this stretch in your hip flexors, abdominals, and chest. To do this stretch, follow these steps:

1. **Stand tall with your feet together, your abdominals and chest lifted, your shoulders back, and your shoulder blades down (see Figure 12-5a).**

2. **Inhale and as you exhale, lunge back with your left leg and reach your left arm up and back (see Figure 12-5b).**

   To feel a deeper stretch in your hip flexor, tuck your pelvis under as you step back.

3. **Inhale and bring your foot and arm back to starting position.**

4. **Repeat this exercise with your right leg and arm.**

5. **Repeat the stretch six to eight more times.**

   As you get stronger, work your way up to two sets of eight.

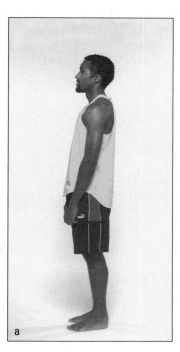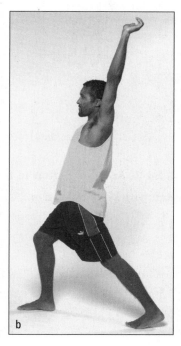

Figure 12-5: The step back lunge with overhead reach.

A few do's and don'ts for this stretch:

✔ Do keep your spine long, even as you reach up and back.

✔ Don't twist or reach to the side.

Triceps stretch

This traditional stretch for the back of your upper arm can be done sitting or standing. To do this stretch, follow these steps:

1. **Stand up tall and raise your left arm and bend your elbow so your fingers are reaching down your spine and your elbow is pointing upward (see Figure 12-6a).**

2. **Place your right hand on your raised elbow, and as you exhale, gently press your elbow back so your fingers of your left hand reach farther down your spine (see Figure 12-6b).**

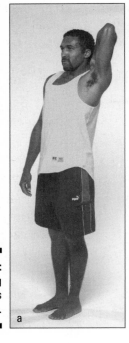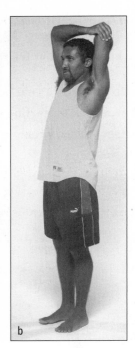

Figure 12-6:
Stretching
your triceps
muscles.

a   b

3. **Hold the stretch for 30 seconds or four to five slow, deep breaths.**

4. **Repeat this stretch with your right arm.**

A few do's and don'ts for this stretch:

- ✔ Do keep your eyes looking forward.

- ✔ Do keep your back straight and deepen the stretch by moving your elbow back, not by arching your back.

- ✔ Don't force or bounce the stretch.

Football

Because of the enormous number and ferocity of the collisions that occur regularly in football, a strong and flexible neck is essential. Coaches and trainers put a lot of time into making sure their athletes' necks are strong and flexible to protect from a severe injury.

Side and back of neck stretch

This stretch is for the muscles that run along the side and back of your neck, down into your upper back. This stretch can be done sitting or standing, but just remember that to effectively stretch this area you must anchor your shoulder blades and keep them still to provide a solid foundation for the stretch.

To do this stretch, follow these steps:

1. **Sit up tall or stand tall with your shoulders down, chest lifted, and abdominals in.**

2. **Exhale and slowly lower your chin toward your chest (see Figure 12-7a).**

3. **Hold this position as you inhale.**

4. **As you exhale, slowly tilt your head to the left, keeping your chin down (see Figure 12-7b).**

   Because the muscles you're stretching attach to your shoulder girdle, you'll diminish the stretch if you raise your shoulders when you tilt your head to the side. Keep your shoulders down.

5. **Inhale again and as you exhale, slightly turn your chin toward your shoulder.**

   This movement is subtle, but you'll definitely feel it in your neck and upper back.

6. **Hold the stretch for one or two more deep breaths and then lift your head back to the center.**

7. **Inhale and lift your shoulders and then exhale as you lower your shoulders.**

8. **Repeat the stretch two to three times and then switch sides.**

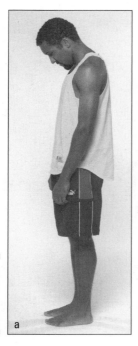
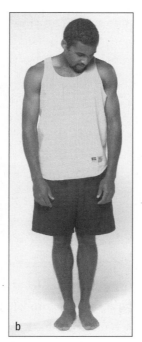

Figure 12-7: Side and back of the neck stretch

A few do's and don'ts for this stretch:

- ✔ Do breathe as you hold the stretch.
- ✔ Do sit up or stand up tall as you hold the stretch.
- ✔ Don't let your shoulders round forward as you drop your head.
- ✔ Don't yank or force the stretch.

Outer thigh stretch

This stretch is for the hip abductors or outer thigh muscles. Because this outer thigh muscle plays an important role in stabilizing your knee, excessively tight hip abductors can cause knee problems because of poor knee alignment. This stretch helps maintain flexibility in your back and trunk area, as well as increases spinal rotation.

To do this stretch, follow these steps:

1. **Sit on the floor with your right leg straight in front of you.**

2. **Bend your left knee and place your left foot on the floor on the outside of your right thigh.**

3. **Inhale and pull your knee toward your chest with your right arm (see Figure 12-8a).**

   Make sure to sit up straight, lengthening your spine.

4. **As you exhale, look over your left shoulder, rotating your spine and tilting your pelvis back (see Figure 12-8b).**

5. **Hold the stretch for 30 seconds, deepening the stretch with every breath.**

6. **Switch sides and repeat the same stretch on your other leg.**

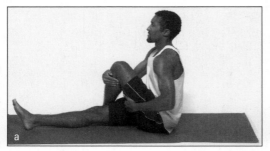 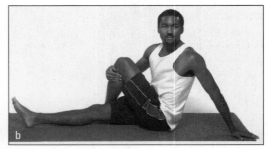

Figure 12-8: Stretching your outer thighs.

A few do's and don'ts for this stretch:

- ✔ Do bring your knee close to your chest before you twist.
- ✔ Do look over your shoulder so you get a lengthening in your neck muscles as well.
- ✔ Do sit up straight to lengthen your spine before you rotate.
- ✔ Don't tuck your pelvis under or round your back.

Swimming

Your deltoid muscle is the primary muscle of your shoulder and is crucial for every swimming stroke there is. Flexibility in this muscle goes a long way toward increasing the range of motion in your stroke and, therefore, your overall speed.

Shoulder stretch with towel or strap

You'll feel this stretch all around your shoulder but particularly in the front part of your deltoid. You need a towel or strap for this stretch — go ahead, run to the closet to get one. I'll wait.

To do this stretch, follow these steps:

1. **Stand up very tall, feet about hip-width apart, holding both ends of a towel or strap in front of your thighs (see Figure 12-9a).**

2. **Inhale, straighten your arms, and raise them overhead (see Figure 12-9b).**

3. **As you exhale, move your arms farther behind your head but don't arch your back (see Figure 12-9c).**

4. **Hold the stretch for 30 seconds or four to five slow, deep breaths.**

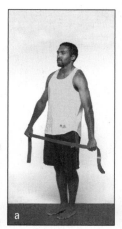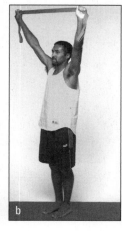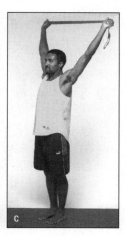

Figure 12-9: Shoulder stretch with towel.

A few do's and don'ts for this stretch:

✔ Do progress through the stretch slowly and gradually.

✔ Do stand up tall as you hold the stretch.

✔ Don't twist to either side.

Deltoid stretch

Range of motion in the shoulder joint is so important for a swimmer. This stretch can be done sitting, standing, or lying down.

To achieve the full effectiveness of the stretch, make sure to maintain good posture.

To do this stretch, follow these steps:

1. **Stand up straight with your feet a comfortable distance apart.**

2. **Contract and lift your abdominals as you gently pull your shoulder blades down.**

3. **Lift your right arm across your chest and hook your other arm under your elbow (see Figure 12-10a).**

   If your shoulders are extremely stiff or tight and you find it difficult to hook your arm underneath your other arm, try the stretch lying on your back. Just drape your arm across your body and let gravity do the work. You may find it more comfortable.

4. **Now, gently lower your right shoulder so it's even with your left shoulder (see Figure 12-10b).**

5. **Inhale and as you exhale, use your left arm to gently pull your right arm across your body.**

6. **Hold the stretch for 30 seconds or four to five slow, deep breaths.**

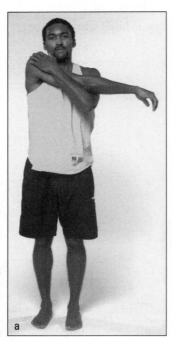 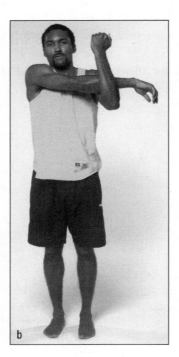

Figure 12-10:
The deltoid stretch.

a   b

A few do's and don'ts for this stretch:

✔ Do breathe as you hold the stretch.

✔ Do progress through the stretch gradually.

✔ Don't pull too forcefully.

Skiing

Skiing requires good coordination, balance, and of course, flexibility to help you move around those large hills of snow! The looser you are when you ski, the more agile you'll be on the slopes.

Standing buttocks stretch

This functional stretch increases your flexibility and strengthens your buttocks muscles while improving your balance and coordination. Use any sturdy surface such as a wall or table to help you stabilize during the stretch.

To do this stretch, follow these steps:

1. **Stand up tall with your ski pole or other supportive surface in front of you.**

2. **Lift your left foot and place it on your right thigh as you slightly bend your right knee.**

3. **Inhale and as you exhale, bend your right knee a little deeper and hinge at your hips so you're hips move back slightly.**

   You should be in a position similar to a squat (see Figure 12-11). You should feel this stretch in your left buttock.

4. **Hold the stretch for 30 seconds or four to five slow, deep breaths.**

5. **Repeat on the other side.**

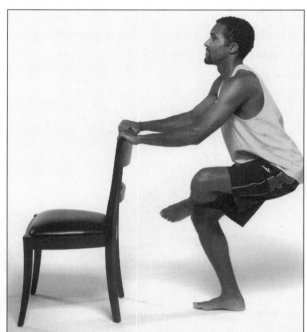

Figure 12-11:
Standing
buttocks
stretch.

A few do's and don'ts for this stretch:

- ✔ Do tilt your pelvis back to feel a deeper stretch in your buttocks.

- ✔ Do keep your back straight and your abdominals lifted.

- ✔ Don't let your knee jut forward. Instead, it should stay directly above your ankle. You should feel your weight mostly in your heel, not in your toes or the ball of your foot.

- ✔ Don't lean too much on your ski pole — it's only there to help you maintain your balance, not to support your body weight.

Lying quad stretch

Skiing really puts a lot of emphasis on your quads. To keep full range of motion in your quads, perform this stretch regularly in the weeks leading up to ski season.

To do this stretch, follow these steps:

1. **Lie on the floor, facedown with both legs straight.**

2. **Rest your forehead on your right fist and bend your left knee and raise your heel toward your buttocks.**

3. **Reach behind you with your left hand and grab the top of your foot and hold your foot in place.**

4. **Inhale and as you exhale, squeeze your buttocks and gently press your left hip toward the floor (see Figure 12-12).**

   Avoid letting your knee move sideways; keep your knees as close together as you can.

5. **Hold the stretch for 30 seconds or four to five slow, deep breaths.**

6. **Repeat the stretch on your right side.**

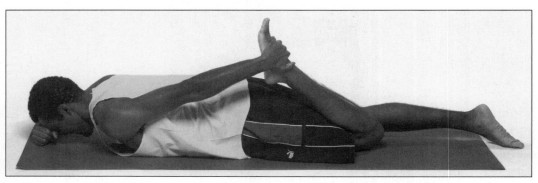

Figure 12-12: Lying quad stretch.

A few do's and don'ts for this stretch:

✔ Do keep your head down, resting on your fist.

✔ Do use your breath to relax into the stretch.

✔ Do keep your knees together and squeeze your buttocks.

✔ Don't focus on bringing your foot to your buttocks, instead focus on pressing your hip toward the floor.

Soccer

Soccer is all about the lower body for both range of motion and endurance. The lower body stretches in this section can be done at the field either before or after your game. Just remember to warm up properly before performing these stretches. See Chapter 11 for some warm-up exercises.

Squat stretch for your inner thighs

Mobility and flexibility are important in the lower body when playing soccer. The following stretch focuses on your groin and inner thigh muscles, as well as your lower back.

Even though the squat can be a very natural and comfortable position, if you experience any pain in your knees due to injury or tightness, discontinue this stretch.

To do this stretch (shown in Figure 12-13), follow these steps:

1. **Begin from a standing position, legs apart and feet slightly turned out.**

2. **Squat down, placing your hands on the floor with your elbows inside your knees.**

   Do keep your feet flat on the floor because that position helps prevent knee strain. If you can't keep your feet flat, you may want to try using a 2 x 4 under your heels.

3. **Hold the stretch for 30 seconds.**

4. **Gently press your elbows against the inside of your knees to deepen the stretch and prevent your knees from rolling inward.**

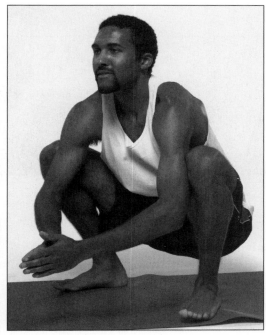

Figure 12-13:
A squat stretch for your inner thigh and groin area.

A few do's and don'ts for this stretch:

- ✔ Do keep knees over your ankles, avoid letting your knees roll inward.
- ✔ Don't tighten or tense your neck and shoulders.

Seated buttocks stretch

Having flexibility in your buttocks may not equate to acceleration in your mind, but it is a little-known fact that your powerful speed can derive from the strength of your buttocks muscles. This stretch helps you get to the ball before the other guy, and look good doing it.

To do this stretch, follow these steps:

1. **Sit on the ground with your right leg straight and the outside of your left ankle on your right thigh, just above your knee.**

   Place your hands behind you to help support your back (see Figure 12-14a).

2. **Inhale and bend your right knee until your right foot is flat on the ground.**

3. **Exhale and lift your chest forward, straightening your back and tilting your tailbone toward the ground (see Figure 12-14b).**

4. **Breathe deeply as you hold the stretch for 30 seconds.**

   Deepen the stretch with each breath by tilting your pelvis back, lifting your chest, and pressing your left knee away from your chest.

5. **Switch sides and repeat the same stretch on your other leg.**

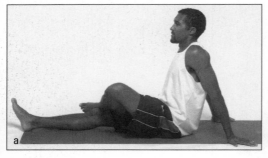 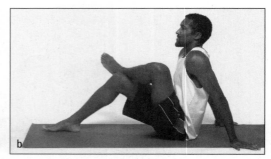

Figure 12-14: Seated buttocks stretch

A few do's and don'ts for this stretch:

- ✔ Do gently hinge forward at your hips.
- ✔ Do keep your back straight, not rounded or tense in your shoulders.
- ✔ Don't look down at your knee; look at the floor in front of your toes.

Cycling

Anyone who's ever ridden a bike knows that the major engine of this sport is the quadriceps muscles. And anyone who's ever ridden a bike for a long time knows how tight the back can get due to the bending over for a long time. The following two stretches address both of these sources of tension.

Supported upper back stretch

Stretching out your tired upper back muscles feels great after a long bike ride.

Make sure to use your bike or any other sturdy support, such as the back of a park bench or a tree during this stretch. And make sure you can place your hands about hip height.

To do this stretch, follow these steps:

1. **Stand with your feet hip-width apart and place your hands on a sturdy surface for support.**

2. **Move your feet back far enough so you can extend your arms as you move your chest toward the floor (see Figure 12-15).**

3. **As you exhale, deepen the stretch by pressing your chest toward the floor and your hips toward the ceiling so you have a slight arch in your back.**

4. **Hold the stretch for 30 seconds or four to five slow, deep breaths.**

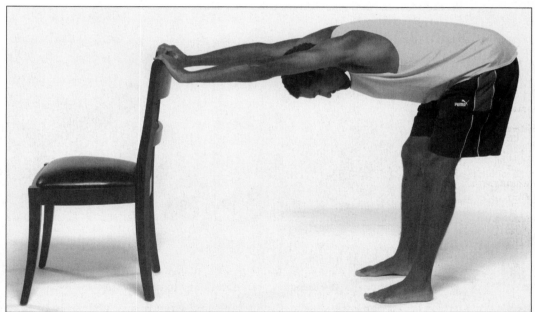

Figure 12-15:
Supported
upper back
stretch.

A few do's and don'ts for this stretch:

✔ Do keep your neck in line with the rest of your spine.

✔ Don't drop your chin to your chest.

✔ Don't round your spine.

Lunging quad stretch

This stretch targets your quadriceps and hip flexors, which can get very tight in cyclists because these muscles are a primary part of the power stroke, especially on long rides.

To do this stretch, follow these steps:

1. **Begin standing, with your legs spread about two feet apart with one foot in front and one foot behind you.**

2. **Inhale and as you exhale, bend both knees and lean forward until you can place both hands on the floor directly behind your front heel.**

3. **Slide your back leg back far enough so you can lower your back knee to the floor without putting weight on your kneecap (see Figure 12-16a).**

4. **Inhale again and as you exhale, gently press your hips toward the floor.**

5. **Inhale and as you exhale, slowly lift your back foot up and grab hold of it with your same side hand (see Figure 12-16b).**

6. **Hold the stretch for 30 seconds or four to five slow, deep breaths.**

7. **Repeat the same stretch on the other side.**

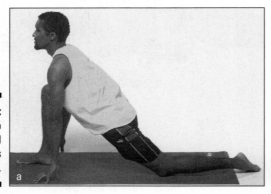 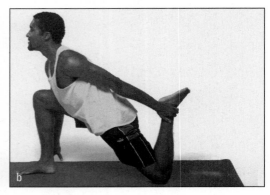

Figure 12-16: Lunging hip flexor and quadriceps stretch.

A few do's and don'ts for this stretch:

- Do keep your chest lifted and your shoulder blades down.
- Do keep your front knee at a right angle and directly over your front heel.
- Don't put your weight on the kneecap of the leg behind you, but instead, your weight should be supported on the softer part of your leg just above your kneecap.

Part IV

Getting Limber As You Live: Stretches for Various Life Stages

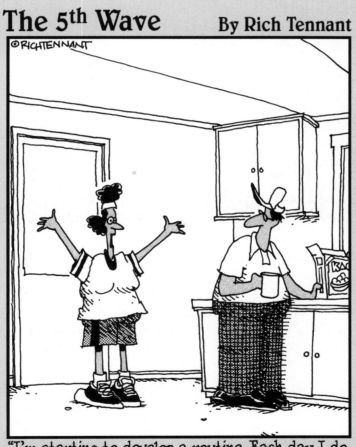

The 5th Wave   By Rich Tennant

"I'm starting to develop a routine. Each day I do some stretches and aerobics, then follow up with high performance nausea and free-style cravings."

In this part . . .

In this part of the book, you discover that no matter what stage of life you're in, stretching can improve your *daily* life. Chapter 13 focuses on pregnancy and contains some of my favorite stretches to help you relax and enjoy this time in your life (Hey, I've had two kids!). Chapter 14 gives you some fun stretches for your kids, no matter what age they are, and Chapter 15 contains a great stretching routine designed to address the concerns of anyone over the age of 60.

Chapter 13

What to Stretch When You're Expecting . . . and After

*I*f you're reading this chapter, you may be pregnant or have just given birth (or interested in the info for someone you know who's pregnant or had a baby — but know that this chapter is directed specifically for mothers to be and new moms). In any case, many discomforts come along with pregnancy and childbirth, and this chapter offers stretching as a way to help! Whether it's swollen feet, a burgeoning belly, or lower back pain, this chapter gives you the best stretching exercises you can do for you and your baby, during pregnancy and after.

How Stretching Can Help if You're Pregnant

When you become pregnant, your body's posture changes in order for the baby to grow, and so your body can get ready for the birthing process. Increased hormones play a big part in these structural changes and allow your ligaments to loosen and stretch. You'll find that some of your muscles tighten while others loosen (my hips got really loose!). As a result, you need to do flexibility exercises for the muscles that get tight.

If you're preggers, here's what stretching can do for you:

✔ Reduce muscle tension in the lower back due to your growing belly

✔ Increase range of movement in the joints

✔ Improve coordination (which you need desperately, thanks to your growing belly)

✔ Aid in the circulation of all the extra blood you have pumping through your veins to various parts of the body

✔ Increase your energy level (a result of increased circulation)

 You may be sitting a lot in the late stages of pregnancy, so take the time to stretch out a bit after you've been sitting in a particular position for a long time. I promise that stretching really helps you keep flexibility in your joints and a bounce in your step! Be good to your body, and it will be good back.

What's happening to your prenatal body?

Oh, who sings that song . . . ChChChCh Changes? Was it the Beatles? I forgot (yet another side effect of pregnancy). And that's exactly what's happening to your body throughout this miraculous time — many, many changes! So take a look at the following list to see what's causing all these changes and why your body's working overtime:

✔ **Fluid retention:** Four to five pounds of your weight gain is from water retention. Your body needs this water to maintain a balance of nutrients for you and the baby.

✔ **Stored fat:** The amount of fat that your body stores varies from four pounds on up, depending on your diet. This element is the one thing of your weight gain that you *can* control, so eating better (not more) while you're pregnant should be your goal.

✔ **Expanding uterus:** Your uterus is expanding to make room for your baby. The uterus weighs two pounds but don't worry, it will tighten and move back into place after the baby is born. In fact, the contractions you feel for a short time after you give birth help squeeze out extra fluid and blood and return the uterus back to its original size.

✔ **Placenta:** The placenta accounts for a one and half pounds of your total weight gain.

✔ **Amniotic fluid:** The *amniotic fluid,* which is the fluid your baby is contained in, makes up two pounds of your baby weight. When your "water breaks," the amniotic sac of fluid is what's actually "breaking."

✔ **Blood volume:** Your blood volume increases approximately 40 percent to support your growing baby. This increase accounts for a total of four pounds. Keeping yourself moving aids in circulation and keeps the oxygen flowing to support the extra weight and the baby within your body.

✔ **Baby:** Six to eight pounds go to the baby, although a lot of women have preemies who weigh around five pounds or babies who weigh well over ten pounds.

✔ **Breasts:** This tissue accounts for two or more pounds.

Stretches for the Pregnant Lady

In this section, I take you through some wonderful pregnancy stretches that help alleviate back pain from carrying all that extra weight around. The following stretches also help counter your loss of balance because that weight gain is all out front!

Pelvic circles

This exercise moves, stretches, and loosens up the hips and pelvis. It also helps ease back pain in late pregnancy and works the glutes and abdominals.

To do this exercise, follow these steps:

1. **Stand with feet hip-width apart and maintain a relaxed bend in your knees.**

2. **Place your hands on your hips (see Figure 13-1a).**

3. **Slowly circle your pelvis ten times clockwise — as if you were using a Hula-Hoop (see Figure 13-2b).**

4. **Repeat the pelvic circle ten times in the opposite direction (counterclockwise).**

A few do's and don'ts for this exercise:

✔ Do keep a slight bend in your knees.

✔ Do place your hands on your hips for balance.

✔ Do breath regularly.

✔ Don't circle your pelvis in too big of circles — keep the movement small.

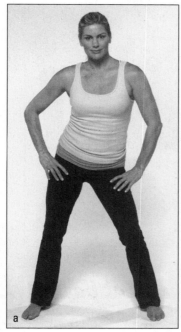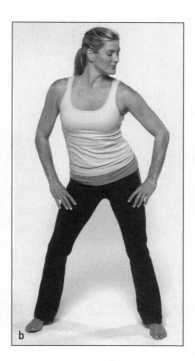

Figure 13-1:
Pelvic circles for looser hips and pelvis.

Extended arm pulse for your upper back

This stretch is great to do during your second trimester and can be done in a sitting position. The movement targets the entire spine and helps relieve upper back pain caused by your growing belly and breasts.

To do this exercise, follow these steps:

1. **Sit on the edge of a chair making sure that your feet are flat on the floor (see Figure 13-2a).**

   Keep your back straight and your abdominal muscles tight and pulled in.

2. **Extend your arms out to your side at shoulder height with your palms facing forward.**

3. **Slowly pulse your arms behind you as if you were trying to squeeze your shoulder blades together (see Figure 13-2b).**

4. **Repeat five times, taking a few slow breaths between stretches.**

A few do's and don'ts for this exercise:

✔ Do keep your feet flat on the floor for balance and support.

✔ Do keep your tummy tight and pulled in.

✔ Don't raise your arms above shoulder level.

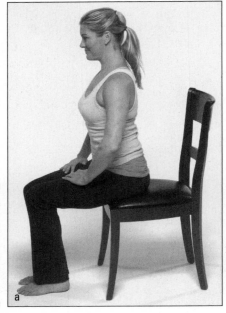 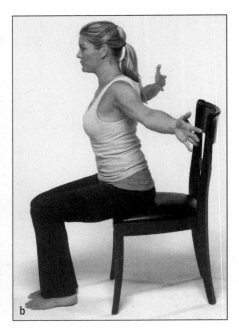

Figure 13-2:
The extended arm pulse stretch for your upper back.

The C-shape that targets your total back

This stretch eases back pain and tension by targeting the muscles in your lower back and stretching out your spine. Be sure to do this stretch whenever you feel lower back discomfort.

To do this exercise, follow these steps:

1. **Stand with your feet hip-distance apart, keeping your knees relaxed (as shown in Figure 13-3a).**

2. **Hold on to a door or stationary object for support, and bend your knees and round your back, tucking your chin toward your chest and tucking your pelvis under (see Figure 13-3b).**

3. **Hold this stretch for ten seconds and repeat several times.**

A few do's and don'ts for this exercises:

✔ Do hold on to something for balance during this stretch.

✔ Do keep your knees slightly bent.

✔ Don't forget to tuck your chin toward your chest to stretch the entire back.

Knee raise for your lower back

This stretch helps relieve lower back pain and the added pressure you may be feeling from weight gain.

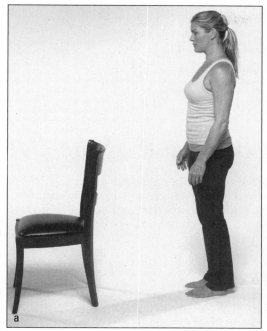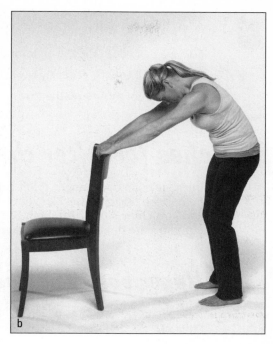

Figure 13-3:
A total back stretch to relieve those tired muscles.

You should only do this stretch in your first trimester because you have to lie on your back, which can decrease blood flow to your baby.

You need a towel to do this stretch.

To do this stretch, follow these steps:

1. **Lie on your back on a mat on the floor, on your bed, or on the couch and bend both knees while keeping your feet flat on the surface you're lying on (see Figure 13-4a).**

2. **Bring your right knee toward your chest and place the towel around your right foot.**

3. **Flex your foot as you gently bring your knee up toward your right shoulder (as shown in Figure 13-4b).**

4. **Hold the stretch for a few seconds and then release.**

5. **Repeat the stretch with your left leg.**

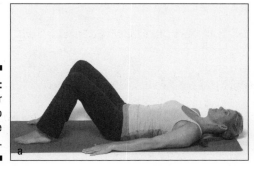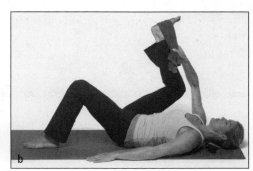

Figure 13-4:
Raising your knees to stretch the lower back.

A few do's and don'ts for this exercise:

- Do flex your foot as you loop the towel around it.
- Do pull the towel gently toward your shoulder.
- Don't forget to breathe through this entire stretch.

Stretches for After the Bun's out of the Oven

Because of all the changes that occurred during labor and delivery, it's going to take a while before you begin feeling like your old self again. So listen to your body and start exercising and stretching slowly. After all, you shouldn't be expected to jump back into the same workout you were doing before you gave birth (or became pregnant).

Upper body stretches

Your upper body gets sore and tight from all the burping and bending over you do when baby arrives (believe me, I just had a baby, and I am sore!). The next two exercises target the shoulders, arms, and chest while increasing circulation to keep the upper body free from tension.

Shoulder reach

This stretch helps relax the shoulders and relieve any soreness you may have in the shoulder joints. To do this exercise, follow these steps:

1. **Sit in a cross-legged position comfortably on the floor with your arms stretched out to the side (see Figure 13-5a).**

2. **Cross your right arm over your chest and hold it with your left hand (as shown in Figure 13-5b).**

3. **Keeping your shoulders relaxed and down, hold the stretch for two breaths and then switch arms.**

Figure 13-5: A shoulder reach to relieve soreness in the joint.

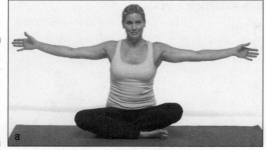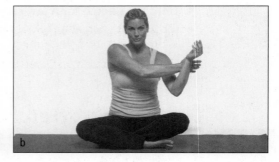

A few do's and don'ts for this exercise:

✔ Do keep your back straight and sit tall during this stretch.

✔ Do inhale as you stretch your arm across your chest.

✔ Don't let your shoulders float up to your neck — keep them pressed down and relaxed.

Chest opener

This stretch feels really good to do after a long day of being hunched over a crib or changing table. The movements open the chest and help relax the upper body.

To do this exercise, follow these steps:

1. **Sit in a comfortable cross-legged position on the floor.**

   Be sure to sit up tall and keep your back nice and straight (as shown in Figure 13-6a).

2. **Inhale as you clasp your hands behind your neck, opening your chest and expanding your lungs (see Figure 13-6b).**

3. **Hold the stretch for two breaths and then release.**

4. **Repeat the movement five times.**

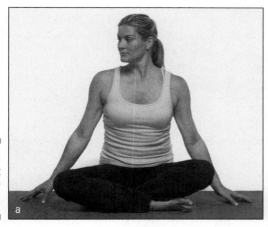 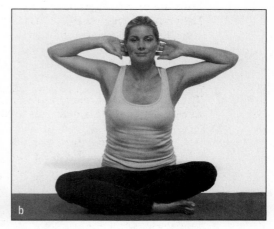

Figure 13-6: The chest opener stretch.

A couple do's and don'ts for this exercise:

✔ Do gaze at the ceiling to help relax your neck and shoulders as you clasp your hands behind your neck and inhale.

✔ Don't arch your back; keep the spine tall and straight.

Lower body stretches

Stretching the lower body is extremely important after giving birth because you spend a lot of time sitting and feeding your baby. Sitting too long can result in tight buttocks muscles and sore hips. The following stretches help relieve these aches and pains that are so common in the lower body.

Lying pelvic tilt

This stretch is a great one for improving lower body circulation and relieving pelvic tension. You can also strengthen the abs, legs, and buttocks with this stretch.

To do this exercise, follow these steps:

1. **Lie on your back with your knees bent and your feet flat on the floor.**

   Your back shouldn't be arched, as shown in Figure 13-7a.

2. **Inhale through your nose, and as you exhale through your mouth gently draw your abdominal muscles in toward your spine (see Figure 13-7b).**

3. **Squeeze your buttocks without lifting your hips.**

4. **Hold for two breaths and then release.**

5. **Repeat Steps 1 through 4.**

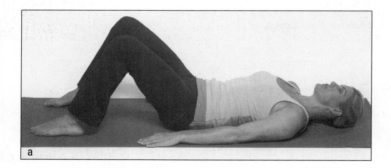

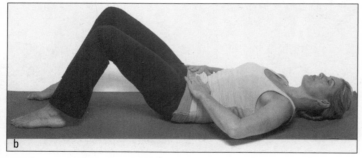

Figure 13-7: Performing the lying pelvic tilt.

A few do's and don'ts for this exercise:

✔ Do keep your feet flat on the floor during this stretch.

✔ Do keep your back flat on the floor to keep from arching.

✔ Don't forget to keep your hands on your abs to feel your muscles tightening.

Kneeling pelvic tilt

By tilting your pelvis toward your spine during this stretch, you're strengthening the abdominal wall as well as stretching out your abdominal muscles. A great stretch for those underused abs!

1. **Get on your hands and knees, making sure to keep your back relaxed and not arched (see Figure 13-8a).**

2. **Inhale and as you exhale, pull your buttocks forward, rotating the pubic bone upward (see Figure 13-8b).**

3. **Hold this position for three seconds and then relax.**

4. **Repeat the stretch five times.**

Figure 13-8: On hands and knees with pelvis in neutral position and then buttocks tucked under.

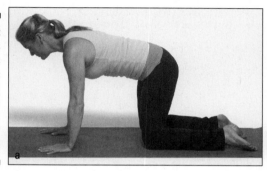 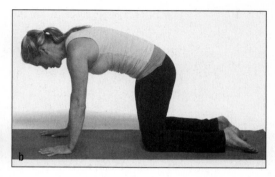

A few do's and don'ts for this exercise:

- ✔ Do keep your back flat and not arched.

- ✔ Do breathe as you pull your pubic bone upward.

- ✔ Don't let your head hang down toward the floor when you're on your hands and knees. Hold it straight and in line with your spine.

Chapter 14

Family Fun: Kid-Friendly Stretches

*Y*ou might think that because school-age kids' muscles are still so new and fresh they would naturally be flexible. But just ask any soccer mom or cheerleading coach and you'll find that the subject of flexibility and children is often misunderstood.

Although very young kids do in fact have naturally pliable muscles and joints, children between the ages of 6 and 12 experience bursts of rapid bone growth at a rate that can actually create tension in the connective tissues that aren't growing as quickly. These spurts result in a surprising tightness in their still very young muscles. So don't be fooled when you see how flexible young gymnasts are on TV, most kids aren't that limber.

Research shows that children need stretching for the same reasons adults need stretching: to help them develop body awareness, increase flexibility, and improve performance in sports. And no matter what age or level of conditioning your children are at, children will exercise if it's presented as play (however if it's presented to them like broccoli, you can forget it!). That's why I've tried to make the stretches in this chapter fun and lighthearted for the little ones, and for the older kids, a little more challenging and useful.

Enticing Children to Get Off Their Tushes

Every advantage you can give your kids, no matter how small, can pay off big in the future. And when it comes to helping them increase their flexibility, it doesn't take a lot to get the job done: A spirited game of Twister may easily do the trick, as does setting limits for the amount of time your kids sit at the computer or play X-Box. Take a break for a little stretching, and tell your kiddos that the break will improve their game score — they'll love it! Or better yet, buy them a hip dance game like "Dance, Dance Revolution." It comes with a dance pad and you actually move your feet, not just your thumbs! Better still, you play it with them!

If your kids like to plop themselves in front of the TV all day, try to come up with some creative movements your children can do while watching TV. Here are some prime examples of TV programming you should use to your advantage:

✔ **Sporting events:** If your kids are watching sports and they see someone warming up in the on-deck circle or on the sideline, point out that every high-level athlete stretches and warms up before getting in the game. Suggest that they try the same move right there in your living room. See how they do. Talk about how it feels. Is it easy? Is it hard? Do they know what muscle they're stretching? Have them show you a move or stretch that their coach (if they play sports) has had them do.

Then the next step is for you to get down on the floor with your little ones and work on your flexibility as a family! The secret is making it fun, and trust me, the kids will get a big kick out of watching Mom or Dad trying to do something difficult — it makes you look surprisingly human. This family time is a good way to exercise your humility and make you more flexible, too!

✔ **Commercial breaks:** While watching their favorite TV show, have your kids stretch during the commercial breaks. Most commercials are about 30 seconds, which is about how long you should hold a stretch. Suggest that your children come up with a different stretch for each commercial and hold it for the duration of the commercial. See who can be the most creative!

To get a jump on this situation, it's important to get kids moving early in their lives. More important, as parents, you need to be healthy role models so your kids grow up *loving* to move. No matter what form of movement you choose to encourage, all that matters is that it should be fun and playful for younger kids and fun and challenging for older kids.

Keep in mind that you are helping to develop crucial attitudes toward fitness, as well as sound workout techniques that last them throughout their lives.

Creative Stretches for 4-to-8-Year-Olds

You can't really expect young kids to hold a hamstring stretch, so you have to do whatever you can to make stretches in general fun and appealing. That's why, in this section, I make the stretches resemble mostly animal movements. At this age, kids love to talk about animals: what they look like, how they move, and what sounds they make.

But remember to keep your stretches and exercises simple — the less complicated the better, especially in the 4- to 8-year-old group. Consider the following ideas for your stretching time:

✔ **Pick a theme** such as animals, dinosaurs, or bulldozers and use your imagination to tell a story about whatever theme you choose.

For example, my child loves animals, so one day we might be a mommy and baby grizzly bear and we need to eat. We walk around the room on our hands and feet pretending to search for food. Sometimes we find food on the ground; sometimes we have to reach into the trees, and sometimes we reach into the water to catch fish. We imagine it is very hot so we move very slowly. After we eat, we are very tired, so we stretch before we lie down. On another day we might be giraffes eating the tops of very tall trees. Whatever the adventure is, we have fun — and the best part is that we stretch not only our bodies, but also our imaginations!

✔ **Play a game** such as "Mother-may-I" or "Hot Potato."

✔ **Use props** such as balls or ribbons on sticks.

For some more good ideas on exercising with your kids, check out the kids' chapter in *Exercise Balls For Dummies* (Wiley) by yours truly or two programs starring Madeleine Lewis: *On the Ball Kit for Ages 3-6* or *On the Ball Kit for Ages 7-10* (both distributed by Gaiam).

For the animal poses in this section, I suggest that you demonstrate them first. Making bizarre animal noises, singing songs, and telling jokes all add to the fun and playful atmosphere — there's no reason to tell your kids that these are really sound and effective stretching exercises.

Reach for the stars!

Your child will have fun using her imagination for this total body stretch. This exercise warms up your kids and stretches them out for the routines later in this chapter (it also helps them count!).

To do this exercise, follow these steps:

1. **Have your child stand very tall with her feet together.**

2. **Explain that there are beautiful stars high above her head and you want her to try to catch ten of them for you (see Figure 14-1a).**

   I tell my daughter to catch ten stars and give them to me before we can start to play games. I ask her to imagine that the stars are very high above her head, so she must reach as high up as she can. Be sure to encourage your child to reach higher and higher as she counts to ten.

3. **After the stars are collected, ask your child to bring them to you.**

   Imagine that you see the stars and tell your daughter how beautiful the stars are. If your child was having fun, ask her to get ten more. Imagine that this time the stars are all over the room and the kids must run and catch them (see Figure 14-1b).

4. **Repeat the stretch two or three times or as long as your kids are having fun!**

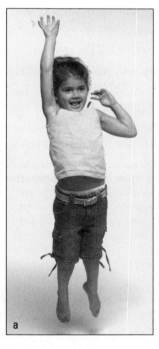 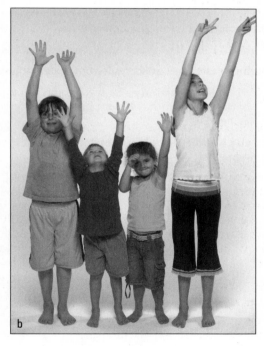

Figure 14-1: Reach for the stars: A fun imaginary game that stretches a child's arms, upper back, and shoulders.

Use this stretch to reinforce knowledge of shapes and colors as well. Instead of having the children find 10 or 15 stars, have them imagine that they have to reach for different color stars, and they have to shout out what color they see. Or explain that different shapes are floating in the air and that they have to call out what they see.

A few do's and don'ts for this exercise:

- ✔ Do make the stretch fun.
- ✔ Do encourage the kids to reach as high as they can, even if it means getting way up on their tiptoes.
- ✔ Do use your imagination and act like you see the stars, too!
- ✔ Don't criticize — there is no right or wrong way to do this exercise.
- ✔ Don't take too long to explain; just get them reaching and then you can go into more detail as they move.
- ✔ Don't rush the kids. If they're enjoying themselves, let them continue playing and reaching.

The seal

Most kids have seen a seal show at a marine park or aquarium, or maybe they've actually been lucky enough to see seals in their natural habitat. Either way, use this memory or image to get the kids to stretch their abdominal muscles and increase flexibility in their spine.

To do this exercise, follow these steps:

1. **Have your child lie on his belly.**
2. **Tell him to raise the upper body up and rest his weight on his elbows.**
3. **Ask him to clap and make noises like a very happy seal (see Figure 14-2).**

   Let your child be as loud as he wants, and reinforce making the sounds, because if your kid is barking, you know he's not holding his breath, and he's getting all the oxygen his muscles need.

4. **Continue barking for about ten seconds and then lower down and pretend to be sleeping seals.**
5. **Repeat the stretch two or three times or as long as your child's having fun!**

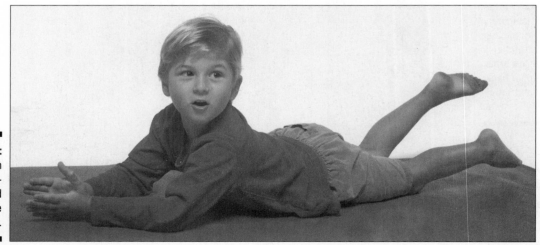

Figure 14-2: Seal stretch for abdominal and spine flexibility.

A few do's and don'ts for this exercise:

✔ Do make the stretch fun!

✔ Do encourage the kids to lift as high as they can without lifting their hips off the floor.

✔ Don't criticize.

✔ Don't rush — let your kids play as seals as long as they want.

The dinosaur walk

Take your kids back to dinosaur times! Ask them to imagine they are turning into a Stegosaurus — not only will they have fun, but also they'll be stretching their calves, hamstrings, back, and shoulders all at once. (You may want to show them a picture of a Stegosaurus so they know what you're talking about — a quick search on the Internet will produce all the pictures you need.)

To do this exercise, follow these steps:

1. **Have your child start with his hands and feet on the floor with his bottom up high in the air (see Figure 14-3).**

2. **Tell your child to imagine that he's turning into a very large Stegosaurus, and ask him to walk slowly forward around the room like a big dinosaur, alternating arms and legs.**

3. **Tell your kid to stop because it's time to take a bite of grass or a drink from a cool pond.**

   As he holds this position and acts out a Stegosaurus drinking or eating, he gets a great stretch without even realizing it.

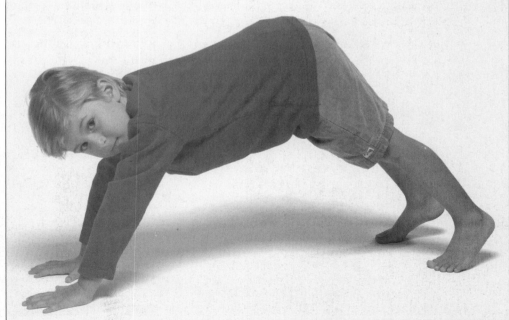

Figure 14-3: Pretending to be a dinosaur helps kids stretch their calves, hamstrings, back, and shoulders.

A few do's and don'ts for this exercise:

✔ Do use your imagination to really playact with the kids.

✔ Do slow the children down if they're walking too fast.

✔ Do walk around the room and see if you can get the kids to lift their hips a little higher or lower their heels to the floor (this tweak helps stretch their calves and hamstrings).

✔ Don't criticize or give too many directions — this exercise should be fun.

The flamingo

Just standing on one leg is a fun challenge for any young child. It's great for their balance and coordination, and here I show you how to turn a simple trick into a flexibility exercise.

To do this exercise, follow these steps:

1. **Ask your child if she has seen flamingos at the zoo, and then ask if she remembers if the flamingos were standing on one leg or two.**

   Explain that flamingos always stand, and to sleep they stand on one leg.

2. **Invite your child to stand on one leg (with the other foot planted on the inside of the standing leg's calf) and pretend to be sleeping flamingos (see Figure 14-4).**

3. **Tell your kid to make snoring sounds as if she were sleeping, and hold the position for 20 to 30 seconds.**

   Snoring promotes breathing in a fun way during the exercise, and it may take your child's mind off trying to stay balanced.

4. **Wake your little flamingo up and have her stand on her other leg and again be a sleeping, snoring flamingo, repeating Steps 1–3.**

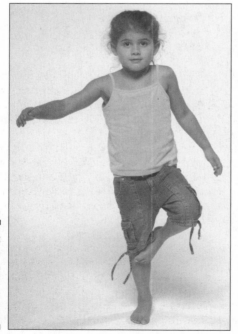

Figure 14-4:
The flamingo provides a fun balance challenge.

Yoga for kids

Imagine that instead of playing softball and basketball during PE in school, kids were asked to take a stab at downward dogs and cobra poses (those are yoga poses). Sounds like a total nonstarter for American kids, right? (Maybe for kids back in the Dark Ages when the baby boomers were trudging through snow to school uphill both ways, but not anymore.)

In a surprising number of schools nationwide, yoga has begun to make an appearance as an addition to — or in a growing number of cases, a substitute for — traditional sports during PE time. Think about it: Yoga requires no expensive equipment; it's accessible to both boys and girls; it requires no large playing fields to maintain; and the incidence of injury is low compared to football or soccer.

Documented benefits are surprisingly numerous and encouraging as well. Across the country teachers, administrators, and happy parents report calmer, more focused students, and in cases where the only difference was the introduction of regular yoga to the curriculum, measurably higher grades — all as a result of doing 5,000-year-old stretching moves and lying quietly for a little while. Looks like 'no pain, no gain' has finally been proven false, once and for all.

A great source of yoga instruction for young ones is any of the titles in Marsha Wenig's *Yoga for Kids* video series (distributed by Gaiam)

After a few intervals of being a flamingo, your child may be ready for more of a challenge. Have her hold on to a wall or sturdy chair with one hand while following the steps for the standing quad stretch in Figure 14-9. This stretch is a little more advanced than just balancing, and it also stretches the front of the thighs a little deeper.

A few do's and don'ts for this exercise:

- ✔ Do focus on the fun and let your little ones giggle and wobble.
- ✔ Don't let the child lift her knee so high behind her that it tilts the hip back, making balancing more difficult.
- ✔ Don't let your child be a slouching flamingo — be a tall, proud flamingo!

Sports Stretches for 9- to 12-Year-Olds

Soccer parents ask me all the time about stretches for their middle-school-age kids. My first reaction is to tell them to have their kids make their beds — leaning out over the mattress to tuck in the sheets and blanket is a great hamstring stretch and kills two birds with one stone! But to be honest, the flexibility needs of kids at this age really require more detailed attention.

Not only can older children follow stretching directions similar to the way adults do, but also their growing bodies have flexibility needs approaching those of adults. For instance, if a young athlete neglects stretching and has tight hamstrings and/or hip flexors, that condition can lead to lower back pain, just like in adults. And, according to the American Academy of Pediatrics, stretching before and after sports increases flexibility, enhances performance, and most important, helps prevent injuries.

Kids tend to be competitive in everything at this age, so enforce the fact that stretching isn't a competition. Your child doesn't have to do the splits just because the friend next door does them. Make sure that your child listens to his body and goes slowly. The stretching program can still be challenging though. Encourage proper form, and try to motivate your child to stretch regularly by tracking results. When he notices that he can run faster or is closer to doing the splits or hitting a home run or achieving any other goal, he'll be more likely to stick with his program.

Keep in mind that the attention span of children in this age group is a little shorter than that of adults. Try to focus on only a few key stretches.

The following stretch routine (all stretches combined make the routine) is designed to address all major muscles groups, and the workout only takes a few minutes. What's more, the following stretches are great for your kids no matter what they do. What really matters is building body awareness and stretching regularly, which helps your kids now, and also in the future.

Butterfly stretch

The butterfly stretch specifically targets the inner thigh and groin. This area is important for kids to stretch because this is a common spot for injuries sustained in active play. I like this stretch for this age group because not only is it fun, but also it is effective and easy to do. It's great in a team sports setting where kids can sit in a circle and face each other and talk while holding the stretch.

Although this stretch is traditionally called the butterfly stretch, kids aren't supposed to flap their knees like a butterfly — that type of move is called *ballistic stretching,* (for more information about the different categories of stretches, see Chapter 1) and you don't want them to do that now. Remember, your goal is to improve kids' flexibility in their inner thigh area, not rip the muscles off the bone.

To do this exercise, follow these steps:

1. **Sit upright on the floor with your knees bent, the soles of your feet touching, and your hands on the floor behind you (see Figure 14-5a).**

   Placing your buttocks against a wall may help you keep your back straight and prevent you from rounding your back.

2. **Place your hands on your feet or ankles and as you inhale, gently pull them as close to your groin as you comfortably can.**

3. **Rest your elbows on your inner thighs, close to your knees.**

4. **As you exhale, lean forward from your hips (see Figure 14-5b).**

   Make sure that you keep your back straight and chest lifted. As you lower your chest toward the floor, also gently press your knees down with your elbows.

5. **Hold the stretch for 30 seconds or four to five slow, deep breaths.**

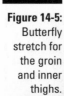

Figure 14-5: Butterfly stretch for the groin and inner thighs.

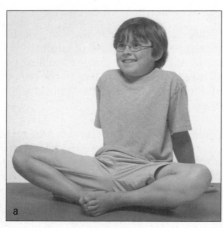
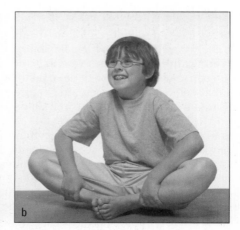

A few do's and don'ts for this exercise:

✔ Do keep your abdominals lifted.

✔ Do keep your shoulder blades down to help keep your chest lifted.

✔ Do think of your spine lengthening, not shortening. Imagine a string attached to the crown of your head pulling you up and forward.

✔ Don't round your back, the movement forward should come from your hips, not your back.

Modified hurdler stretch

Tight hamstrings can have a negative effect on your child's ability to kick, run, and jump by reducing their range of motion and exposing them to the risk of injury. So whether your child plays a team sport or racquet sport, does gymnastics, takes dance classes, or just likes to run around the playground, having flexibility in the hamstrings is an advantage.

Use a towel with this stretch; it helps you keep your back straight while you lean forward. If you can keep your back straight, you'll have a better chance of stretching your hamstrings (the back of your thighs) without straining your lower back.

To do this stretch, follow these steps:

1. **Sit on the floor with your right leg straight and your left leg bent so the sole of your foot is flat against the inside of your right knee.**

2. **Place a towel around the ball of your right foot and hold on to both ends of the towel (see Figure 14-6a).**

3. **As you exhale, hinge forward at the hip and gently pull on the towel to help you lean forward without rounding your back (see Figure 14-6b).**

   Imagine your tailbone moving toward the back of the room and the heel of your straight leg reaching toward the front of the room. This position should lengthen the back of your leg from both directions. Your tailbone should be reaching back as you hinge forward at the hips. Remember to keep the knee straight.

4. **Breathe deeply as you hold the stretch for 30 seconds.**

   Deepen the stretch with each breath by tilting your pelvis back, lifting your chest, and flexing your foot so your toes are moving toward your shoulders.

5. **Switch sides and repeat the same stretch on your other leg.**

   Don't get discouraged if your chest is nowhere near your leg. As long as you're feeling a good deep stretch in the back of your thigh, and you're keeping your back straight, then you're doing great!

Figure 14-6: Modified hurdler stretch with a towel or strap.

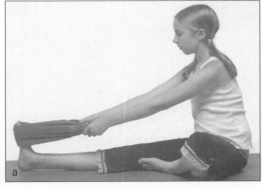
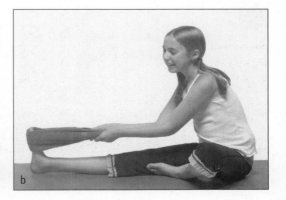

A few do's and don'ts for this stretch:

- ✔ Do gently hinge forward at your hips.
- ✔ Do keep your knee straight, and try to keep the back of your knee on the floor.
- ✔ Do keep your back straight, not rounded or tense in your shoulders.
- ✔ Don't look down at your knee; look at the floor in front of your toes.

Straddle stretch

This is my favorite stretch to help you achieve a perfect split!

To do this stretch, follow these steps:

1. **Sit up tall with your hands behind you for support and your legs straight out in front of you.**

2. **Open your legs and move your feet away from each other (see Figure 14-7).**

   You should feel the stretch along your inner thighs.

3. **Hold the stretch for 30 seconds or for four to five slow, deep breaths.**

To deepen the stretch you can place your hands on the inside of your thighs and gently press your legs a little wider. Also, placing a small rolled towel under your hips can intensify the stretch.

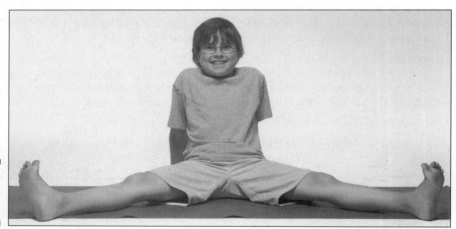

Figure 14-7:
Straddle
stretch.

A few do's and don'ts for this stretch:

- ✔ Do progress through the stretch gradually and slowly.
- ✔ Don't bounce or force the stretch.

Runner's lunge

The runner's lunge is one of the best stretches for anyone, not just for a runner. The exercise targets three small hip muscles, which are called your iliopsoas or hip flexors. This area can get very tight if you engage in sports, because the hip flexors are the muscles that lift your knee or move your leg forward, such as kicking or walking or running or just about anything that has to do with forward motion. Ironically, these muscles can also get tight and shorten if you've been sitting at school all day.

To do this stretch, follow these steps:

1. **Begin by standing with your feet spread about two feet apart, one foot in front and one foot behind you.**

2. **Inhale and as you exhale, bend both knees until you can place both hands on the floor directly behind your front heel (see Figure 14-8a).**

3. **Slide your rear foot back so you can lower your rear knee to the floor without putting weight on that back knee cap (see Figure 14-8b).**

4. **Inhale again, and as you exhale, gently press the front of the hip of the back leg toward the floor.**

5. **Hold the stretch for 30 seconds or four to five slow, deep breaths.**

6. **Repeat the same stretch on the left side.**

If this stretch is uncomfortable for you to get into, try doing it sitting on the edge of an exercise bench to support your body weight with the thigh of the bent leg. Extend your back leg behind you with the ball of your foot on the floor.

Figure 14-8: Runner's lunge for the front of your hip.

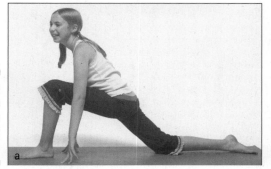 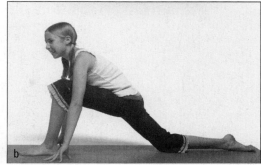

A few do's and don'ts for this stretch:

✔ Do keep your chest lifted and your shoulder blades down.

✔ Do keep your front knee at a right angle directly over your front heel.

✔ Don't jut your front knee forward, which places undue strain on your knee.

✔ Don't put your weight on the kneecap of the leg behind you — your weight should be supported on the softer part of your leg just above your kneecap.

Standing quad stretch

This is a great standing stretch that targets your quads (the muscles in the front of your thigh). This practical and convenient stretch is great to do after you've been exercising outdoors because you stand up to perform it.

To do this stretch, follow these steps:

1. **Stand up tall and place your right hand on a stable surface.**

   This surface can be a chair, wall, doorway, or fence — anything that's sturdy and helps you keep your balance as you put your weight on one leg.

2. **As you inhale, lift your left knee forward and grab your ankle or top of your foot with your left hand (see Figure 14-9a).**

3. **As you exhale, slowly lower your knee until it's even with the knee of the standing leg (see Figure 14-9b).**

4. **Gently support the foot behind you with your hand.**

   Focus on moving your knee back, not yanking your foot up to touch your buttocks. Try to keep the inside of your thighs touching. To really feel this stretch correctly, try to tuck your pelvis under and think about your tailbone moving toward the floor.

5. **Hold the stretch for 30 seconds or four to five slow, deep breaths.**

   Have fun and try to make this a balance exercise as well. As you are holding the stretch, try to let go of the stable surface and see if you can hold your balance as you continue to stretch your quadriceps.

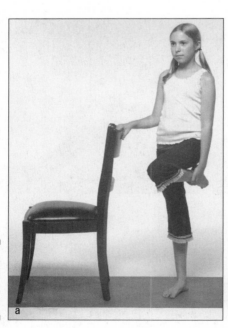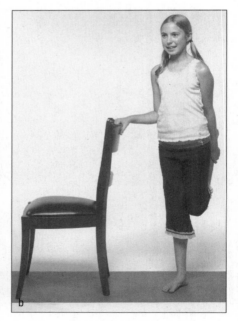

Figure 14-9:
Standing quad stretch.

A few do's and don'ts for this stretch:

✔ Do stand up tall with your chest lifted, abs in, and shoulder blades down. This position helps you feel the stretch correctly and practices good posture!

✔ Don't put undue stress on your knee by forcing your foot up to touch your buttocks.

✔ Don't let your bent knee move to the side; keep the insides of your legs touching.

Reaching down your back, elbows high

This traditional stretch for the back of your upper arm (your triceps) can be done sitting or standing. To do this stretch, follow these steps:

1. **Stand up tall and raise your left arm and bend your elbow so your fingers are reaching down your spine and your elbow is pointing upward (see Figure 14-10a).**

2. **Place your right hand on your raised elbow, and as you exhale, gently press your elbow back so your fingers of your left hand reach farther down your spine (see Figure 14-10b).**

3. **Hold the stretch for 30 seconds or four to five slow, deep breaths.**

4. **Repeat this stretch with your right arm.**

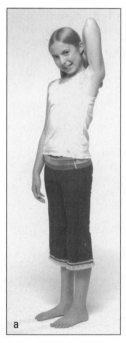
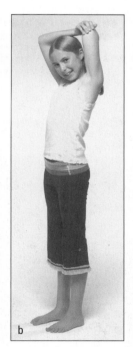

Figure 14-10: A triceps stretch.

a

b

A few do's and don'ts for this stretch:

✔ Do keep your eyes looking forward.

✔ Do try to walk your fingertips farther down your back.

✔ Don't arch your back.

✔ Don't force or bounce the stretch.

Shoulder pull

The deltoid muscle is the muscle that wraps around the top of your shoulder joint. You use it every time you lift your arm, so no matter what sport or activity you engage in, you probably use this muscle a lot.

Having flexibility in your shoulder helps you swing a baseball bat better, improves your stroke in tennis, and gives you a more powerful golf swing. This stretch can be done sitting, standing, or lying down.

To do this stretch, follow these steps:

1. **Stand up tall with your feet flat on the floor and your abdominals lifted.**

2. **Lift your right arm horizontally across your chest, and hook your left arm outside your elbow (see Figure 14-11a).**

3. **Gently lower your right shoulder so it's even with your left shoulder and use your left arm to gently pull your right arm across your body (see Figure 14-11b).**

5. **Hold the stretch for 30 seconds or four to five slow, deep breaths.**

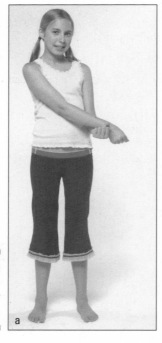
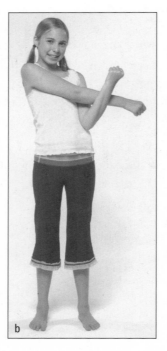

Figure 14-11: The shoulder pull for the deltoid.

a

b

If your shoulders are extremely stiff or tight and you find it difficult to hook your arm over your other arm, try doing this stretch lying on your back. Just drape your arm across your body and let gravity do the work. You may find it more comfortable.

A few do's and don'ts for this stretch:

- ✔ Do progress through the stretch gradually.
- ✔ Do stand up or sit up tall as you hold the stretch.
- ✔ Don't let your shoulder lift or kink your neck.
- ✔ Don't pull too forcefully.

Backward arch on a ball

You'll love this stretch because it's done on one of those large exercise balls, which adds a fun element of balance. This stretch is mainly for the muscles of your chest, but it's also a great stretch for your abs.

If you have never used an exercise ball before, take a few minutes initially to get used to it. At first it may seem difficult to keep your balance, but you'll get use to it very fast. If you still feel wobbly, you can perform this stretch next to a wall or exercise bench.

To do this stretch, follow these steps:

1. **Sit upright on the ball.**
2. **Walk your feet two or three steps forward so you roll down on the ball to the point where your shoulder blades are supported against the ball and your spine is in neutral position.**
3. **Interlock your hands behind your head (see Figure 14-12a).**
4. **Inhale deeply and as you exhale, slowly lower your head toward the ball, letting your elbows drop toward the sides of the ball (see Figure 14-12b).**

   You should feel this stretch in the upper chest area.
5. **Hold this stretch for 30 seconds and then release by lifting your head and walking your feet back until you're sitting upright on the ball again.**

   This stretch may feel so good that you may want to do it again, but you don't have to.

If you like this stretch, check out other stretches using the ball in my book *Exercise Balls For Dummies* (Wiley). It's full of fun exercises, using a ball to both strengthen and stretch your entire body.

A few do's and don'ts for this stretch:

- ✔ Do relax your neck and shoulders.
- ✔ Do keep your shoulder blades on the ball.
- ✔ Don't bounce your elbows up and down.
- ✔ Don't hold your breath!

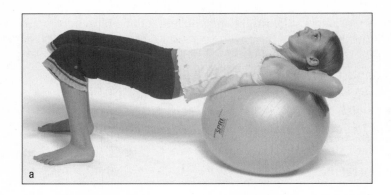

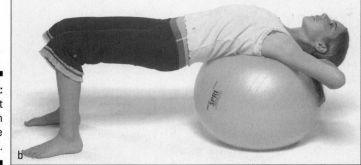

Figure 14-12:
Chest
stretch on
an exercise
ball.

Chapter 15

Seventh Inning Stretch: Special Stuff for Seniors

- -

In This Chapter

▶ Figuring out your exercise limitations

▶ Stretching to increase your flexibility

- -

*I*t's an unavoidable fact of life that flexibility diminishes with age. Studies paint a pretty bleak picture: Over time, range of motion decreases in the neck, shoulders, back, hips, ankles, and wrists. In other words, as you get older you lose range of motion in just about every movement you make. This loss can affect a wide variety of everyday functions, such as tying your shoes, reaching for something on the top shelf, or turning around in your car to back out of the driveway.

Stretching, however, is a simple and powerful weapon to help you fight the debilitating effect of the passing years. Research has proven that stretching can significantly improve flexibility in the older adult, which means that you *don't* have to give in to the increasingly rust in your joints.

Regular stretching is without a doubt one of the most important things you can do to keep your body functioning as smoothly as possible. Stretching can't turn back the clock, but it can slow it down considerably.

Determining Your Limits and Recognizing Changes

People over age 65 represent the most rapidly growing group in the population (welcome, baby boomers!). But the characteristics of the people in this age group can vary wildly because of the many different degrees of health and fitness of individuals in this age range. So it would be incorrect to consider everyone over 65 as one group. Nevertheless, when it comes to stretching, a couple of age-related factors go across the board:

✔ **Your range of motion is smaller than it used to be.** Because age-related changes in muscle structure can lead to increased muscle stiffness, if you're just starting a flexibility program, your range of motion may be quite limited. To help determine your present range of motion, see the Flexibility Self-Evaluation Worksheet in Chapter 3.

In light of your lessened range of motion, in order not to place too much stress on already stiff muscles and joints, I recommend holding the stretches in this chapter for a shorter amount of time than I regularly do, and then repeating the stretch. For example, instead of holding a stretch for 30 seconds, hold it for 15 seconds, relax, and then repeat the stretch. As you get more flexible, you may want to then begin to hold the stretches for longer; it's all about listening to your body!

✔ **Maintaining your balance isn't so easy anymore.** For this reason, I added a few props for the following stretches, such as a chair or wall, to help add stability to each stretch.

✔ **Medical issues are more of a concern.** Take into account any preexisting medical issues you may have, such as osteoporosis or arthritis, and discuss them with your doctor. One good rule of thumb is that you should always feel better after stretching, not worse.

A Stretch Routine to Help You Maintain Flexibility

The following stretches are specifically designed to be accessible to anyone — even someone with physical limitations due to age or injury. None of these moves requires you to get down on the ground or to assume complicated positions. This full-body routine is simple and straightforward and helps increase your range of motion from your head to your toes.

Back and shoulders stretch

Loss of range of motion and flexibility in the shoulders and back can create functional limitations in this area. Performing this stretch every day can help you maintain and even increase range of motion in your shoulders and back.

To do this stretch, follow these steps:

1. **Stand behind a chair and place your hands on the top of the chair.**

2. **Walk backward until your arms are straight and your knees are slightly bent. Keep your feet shoulder-width apart (see Figure 15-1a).**

3. **Inhale and as you exhale, let your chest sink toward the floor until you feel the stretch in your shoulders and back.**

   Keep your head level between your arms. Your eyes should be looking at the floor, not at your shoes (see Figure 15-1b).

4. **Hold the stretch for a few deep breaths or as long as is comfortable.**

5. **Walk your feet back toward the chair, slowly rounding your back until you're upright.**

6. **Inhale and repeat the stretch one more time.**

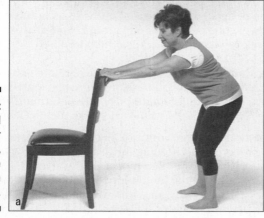 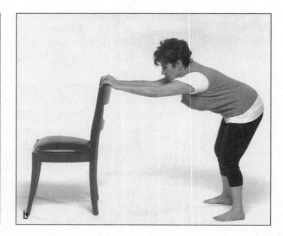

Figure 15-1: Back and shoulder stretch, using the support of a chair.

A few do's and don'ts for this stretch:

- ✔ Do keep your shoulder blades down and your upper body relaxed.
- ✔ Do keep your back straight, not rounded.
- ✔ Don't bounce or force the stretch; keep it gentle and slowly progress into a deeper stretch.

Standing side reach with chair for support

Using the back of a chair for support in the standing side reach stretch allows you to deepen the stretch without risking losing your balance or reaching too far. Feel the stretch in your shoulders, back, abs, and even the top part of your hip.

To do this stretch, follow these steps:

1. **Stand with the back of your chair about a foot from your right side.**
2. **Place your right hand on the top of the back of the chair.**
3. **Stand with your feet about 12 to 14 inches apart, your knees slightly bent, and your toes forward (see Figure 15-2a).**
4. **Inhale and reach your left arm directly overhead with your palm facing inward.**

   Use the muscles in your upper back to keep your shoulder blade down. This should keep space between your shoulder and ear.
5. **As you exhale, lean to the right, keeping your right hand on the back of the chair for support and your hip and leg anchored to the floor (see Figure 15-2b).**
6. **Hold this stretch for 30 seconds or four to five slow, deep breaths.**
7. **Repeat on the other side.**

If you notice tension in your shoulders, instead of reaching with a straight arm, keep your elbow bent. The movement should come from your waist, not your shoulder.

A few do's and don't for this stretch:

- ✔ Do keep your shoulders and hips facing forward and your knees slightly bent.
- ✔ Do breathe through the stretch.
- ✔ Don't hold the stretch if you feel tension or pain.

Figure 15-2:
Standing
side reach
with chair.

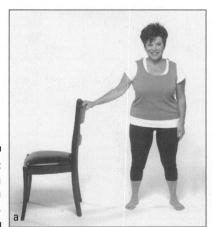
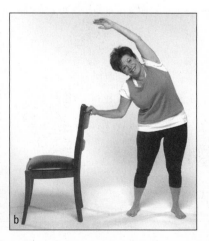

Seated hamstring stretch

The hamstrings (back of the thigh) are one of the tightest muscle groups for most people — no matter what age you are. That's why it's so important to stretch the muscles of the lower body regularly.

Make sure you're in a chair without wheels, or else you'll end up doing a headstand, whether you like it or not. It's important that the chair is sturdy and stable.

To do this stretch, follow these steps:

1. **Sit on the edge of the seat of your chair and extend your left leg straight out in front of you.**

2. **Flex your foot so your toes are moving toward you (see Figure 15-3a).**

3. **Keep your opposite leg bent with your foot flat on the floor and your knee at a 90-degree angle.**

4. **Inhale and sit up very straight, lengthening your spine.**

5. **As you exhale, slowly hinge at your hips and lean forward, tilting your hipbones forward and your tailbone back toward the back of the chair (see Figure 15-3b).**

6. **Hold the stretch for 30 seconds, deepening the stretch with every breath.**

7. **Switch sides and repeat the same stretch on your other leg.**

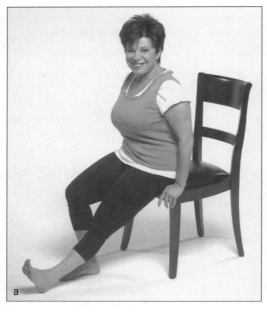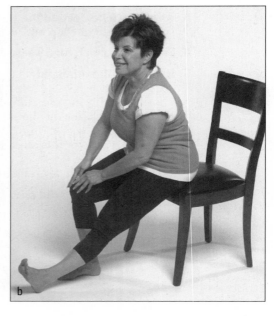

Figure 15-3: Seated in a chair with one leg extended for a hamstring stretch.

A few do's and don'ts for this stretch:

✔ Do sit on the edge of the chair.

✔ Do keep your back straight at all times.

✔ Don't tuck your pelvis under or sit on the cushy part of your buttocks.

Seated inner thigh and groin stretch

The inner thigh and groin area is often difficult to stretch if you have tight hamstrings or back muscles. By performing this stretch sitting in a chair, you'll be able to isolate the inner thigh more effectively and stretch this area without putting stress or strain on your back.

To do this stretch, follow these steps:

1. **Sit on the edge of your chair with your feet flat on the floor.**

2. **Separate your knees as far apart as possible and make sure you sit up tall with your back straight (see Figure 15-4a).**

   Your toes should be slightly pointing outward.

3. **Place your elbows on the inside of your knees and gently push outward as you exhale (see Figure 15-4b).**

4. **Hold for about 30 seconds or four to five slow, deep breaths.**

5. **Repeat the stretch on your other leg.**

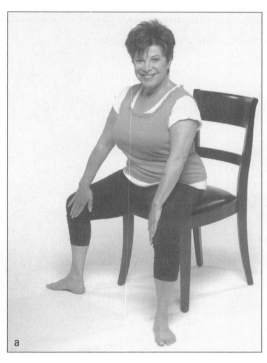 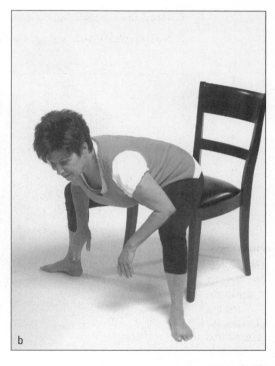

Figure 15-4:
Seated inner thigh and groin stretch.

A few do's and don'ts for this stretch:

✔ Do progress through the stretch gradually.

✔ Do keep your back straight and your shoulder blades down.

✔ Don't bounce or force your knees to go wider.

Seated hip flexor and quadriceps stretch

Tight hip flexors are often the cause of lower back pain. This handy stretch can target this area without even getting out of your chair.

To do this stretch, follow these steps:

1. **Sit close to the front edge of the chair and turn your body to face left and hold on to the back of the chair with your left hand.**

2. **Reach your right foot back, allowing your right knee to move toward the floor (see Figure 15-5a).**

3. **Tuck your pelvis slightly under by squeezing your buttocks of the back leg (see Figure 15-5b).**

4. **Inhale and exhale as you hold for 15 to 30 seconds.**

5. **Repeat this stretch on the other leg.**

Because you're so close to the edge of the chair it's important to never let go of the back of the chair with your hand because you may fall off.

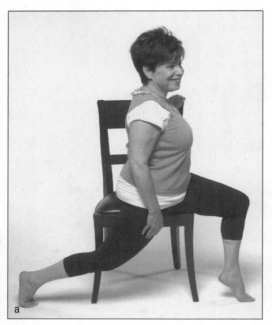 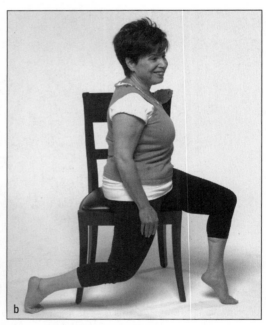

Figure 15-5:
Seated hip flexor stretch.

A few do's and don'ts for this stretch:

- ✔ Do breathe as you hold the stretch.
- ✔ Do hold on to the back of the chair.
- ✔ Do turn your body completely to the side.
- ✔ Do keep your shoulders directly above your hips.
- ✔ Don't round or bend forward at your waist.

Seated spinal rotation

This stretch is excellent to increase the rotational movement in your spine, which in turn may help you back out of the driveway easier!

To do this stretch, follow these steps:

1. **Sit up tall on a sturdy chair with your feet flat on the floor and close together, knees at a right angle.**

2. **Anchor your left hand on the back of the chair as you place your right hand on the outside of your left thigh (see Figure 15-6).**

3. **Inhale and as you exhale, twist your torso to the left and look back over your shoulder.**

4. **Hold the stretch for about ten seconds.**

   Try to make a mental note of a stationary object you see that's about at eye level.

5. **Release the stretch and come back to center.**

6. **Inhale again and as you exhale, repeat the stretch on the same side.**

   Find the same object you were looking at, but this time try to find another object that's past it.

7. **Repeat the stretch series on the opposite side.**

A few do's and don'ts for this stretch:

✔ Do keep your feet flat on the floor.

✔ Do keep your knees and feet together and facing the front.

✔ Don't force the stretch or pull too hard on the back of the chair.

✔ Don't look down — find an object that's at eye level.

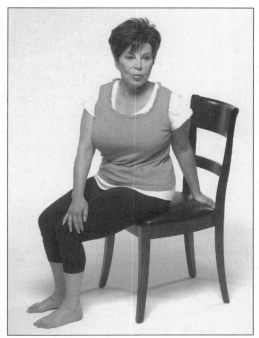

Figure 15-6:
Seated spinal rotation.

Wrist and forearm stretch

Keeping flexible in your hands and wrists is important because a common attribute of the aging process is a decrease in grip strength and a loss of small-motor dexterity — both of which can be helped by this stretch. You'll feel a stretch in the muscles of your wrists, hands, and forearm.

To do this stretch, follow these steps:

1. **Sit tall in your chair with your back straight and your feet flat on the floor.**

   Your shoulders should be relaxed and your abdominals lifted.

2. **Inhale and extend your right arm forward about shoulder height with the palm up.**

3. **As you exhale, grab your fingers with your left hand and gently pull your fingers back toward your body (see Figure 15-7a).**

4. **Release the stretch and rotate your arms so the palm of your hand is facing downward.**

5. **Inhale and use your left hand to gently press your palm toward your body (see Figure 15-7b).**

6. **Hold this stretch for 10 to 15 seconds, breathing deeply throughout the stretch.**

7. **Repeat with the other arm.**

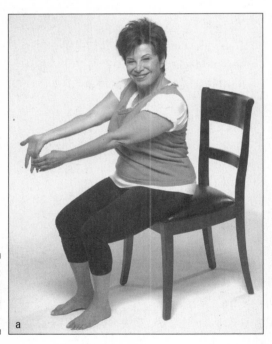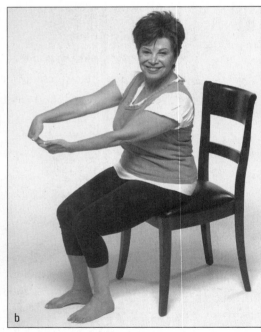

Figure 15-7: Wrist and forearm stretch.

A few do's and don't for this stretch:

✔ Do sit up tall with your feet flat on the floor.

✔ Do keep your arms extended as you stretch the wrist.

✔ Don't bounce or force the stretch.

Seated chest and front of shoulder stretch

Tight chest muscles and weak upper back muscles oftentimes cause excessive rounding of the shoulders. Try this exercise to stretch out your chest and shoulders.

To do this stretch, follow these steps:

1. **Sit up tall on the front edge of a chair.**

2. **Reach behind your back with both arms and link your forearms (see Figure 15-8).**

3. **Inhale and as you exhale, squeeze your shoulder blades together.**

   After several deep breaths, try to deepen the stretch by grabbing your opposite elbow with your hands (see Figure 15-8).

4. **Hold the stretch for about 30 seconds or four to five slow, deep breaths.**

5. **Repeat the same stretch with the other hand on top.**

If your range of motion is limited in your shoulders, and/or you feel pain or discomfort, try performing this stretch one arm at a time. Instead of grabbing both elbows at the same time, reach only one arm across the midline of your back and with your other hand grab hold of your wrist or forearm.

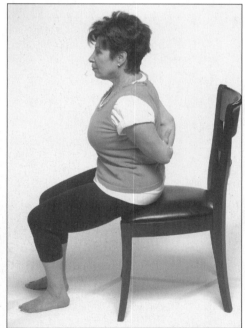

Figure 15-8:
Seated
shoulder
and chest
stretch.

A few do's and don'ts for this stretch:

✔ Do keep your eyes looking forward.

✔ Do maintain good posture throughout the stretch.

✔ Don't let your back arch when you squeeze your shoulder blades together.

Got arthritis?

People used to believe that if they had arthritis they shouldn't exercise, but now exercise has become an important part of treating the disease. Why? Because if you don't take care of the muscles that surround the joint, range of motion will be lost and stiffness and pain increase. The goal of people with arthritis should be to limit the progression of the existing damage in the affected joint or joints, which is most effectively accomplished by strengthening and stretching the muscles that surround the joints. The million dollar question, however, is how much exercise should you do if you're diagnosed with arthritis? Generally, if you have a flare-up in a joint, that's the time to rest and let your medication do its job. As the inflammation decreases and the pain subsides, you can gradually return to exercise. The key word is *gradually*. If you experience pain, that's your cue to stop.

Part V
The Part of Tens

The 5th Wave   By Rich Tennant

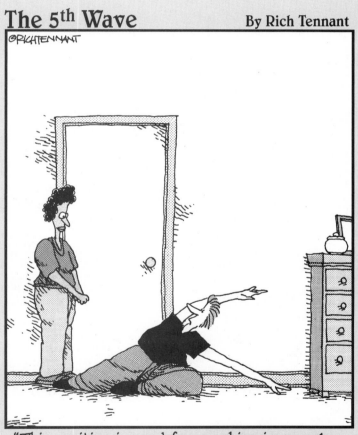

"This position is good for reaching inner calm, mental clarity, and things that roll behind the refrigerator."

In this part . . .

The *For Dummies* crew has a hallowed tradition of ending each book with a top-ten list, and in this book, I end with two of them. In Chapter 16, I list ten common aches and pains that stretching can help minimize or, in some cases, actually prevent, and in Chapter 17, I show you ten simple household items that can be great props to help you get more out of stretching.

Chapter 16

Ten Common Aches and Pains and Stretches that Can Help

. . . .

In this Chapter

▶ Listening to your body's pains
▶ Stretching away the pain

. . . .

Stretching can help create a balance between strength and flexibility, between opposing muscle groups, between your left and right side, and between your mind and body (that's what's meant by "mind, body connection"). Stretching can also help solve many of the mechanical problems that create discomfort. Think of this balance as an organic pain reliever, returning your body to its natural, pain-free state.

In this chapter, I cover ten signals from your body that parts of it may be out of balance. Pain is your body's way of telling you there's a problem that needs to be fixed. I suggest that, in addition to all the tried-and-true methods of pain relief you're used to — like warm soaks and ice-cold packs — you consider stretching as a new, powerful tool in your pain relief arsenal. Instead of reaching for that bottle of anti-inflammatory medication *first* to mask the problem, try a stretch or two.

Stretching is only *one* tool in the battle against pain, so if any of the conditions in this chapter persist for longer than a couple of days, please consult your healthcare professional.

Bursitis and/or Tendonitis

Overuse injuries such as bursitis and tendonitis are the result of irritation within a joint (whether from injury or misalignment) that causes inflammation. *Bursitis* is an inflammation of the *bursa* — a type of connective tissue that cushions tendons and thereby helps prevent friction between the tendon and the bone.

Bursitis can be caused by repetitive motion, or by compression, such as someone who sleeps only on one side or wears tight shoes. *Tendonitis,* which is inflammation of the tendon where the normal smooth gliding motion of the muscle disappears, is caused by excessive use of a tendon, which can lead to microscopic tears in the collagen that makes up the tendon. Either of these conditions can produce a painful irritation of the bursa, and the result is pain and swelling.

The best prevention against these painful conditions is to keep the muscles around your joints strong and flexible to guard against any irritation occurring in the first place. Exercising at least three times a week helps keep your muscles strong, but you also need to keep your joints flexible. Gentle stretches keep the muscles stretchy, which can help keep the pressure and pain away.

The weekend warrior

Many people like to play recreational sports or do home improvement projects on the weekends. And face it; sometimes the weekend is the only time you have to do it. So bursitis and tendonitis are common complaints of weekend warriors because of the repetitive movements involved in some sports and the lack of strength training and stretching during the week. The areas that most commonly become inflamed are the shoulders, elbows, knees, hips, ankles, and heels. If this sounds like something you may be experiencing, I recommend sport-specific stretches, such as those found in Chapter 12. Those stretches help prevent tightness and keep the muscles around the joints you use the most flexible, which leads to a reduction in tension on your tendons from tight muscles and less inflamed bursa. Always stretch at least five to ten minutes after your activity, paying specific attention to the muscles you just worked.

 Nevertheless, if you're already in pain, the first thing you need to do is rest. Wait a few days; after the pain goes away, you can safely begin to stretch the affected area.

 If you suffer from joint pain as a result of arthritis, see Chapter 15 for some simple stretches to help ease the pain. The stretches in Chapter 15 are designed for seniors, but if you have arthritis at any age, those exercises will help relive your pain, too.

Carpal Tunnel Syndrome

Carpal tunnel syndrome is a painful progressive condition caused by compression of a key nerve in the wrist. Symptoms usually start gradually with pain, weakness, or numbness in the hand and wrist and then radiate up the arm. As symptoms worsen, people may feel tingling during the day, and decreased grip strength may make it difficult to form a fist, grasp small objects, or perform other manual tasks.

If you have a job where you sit at your computer all day or you perform some type of repetitive motion with your hands, I suggest the wrist and forearm stretches in Chapter 4. Perform those exercises several times a day as you take short little breaks from your job. These stretches can play an important role in preventing carpal tunnel syndrome.

Indigestion

The causes of indigestion are many, but the solutions are few. Stretching can enhance the digestive process by massaging the intestines and initiating muscular contractions in the abdominal area, both of which can help move things along in there. Stretching is very effective in helping to reduce stress, which in turn calms your stomach.

But one cause of indigestion in particular is stress (see Chapter 10 for information on stress and how it affects your body). Studies have shown that, in men, the "fight-or-flight" response, instigated by stress, restricts blood flow to the abdomen, reduces the production of digestive enzymes, and slows the digestive process overall. These conditions result in bloating, heartburn, and constipation.

Check out the "Stress" section later in this chapter, too.

Insomnia

Insomnia is the chronic inability to fall asleep or remain asleep for an adequate length of time. In many cases, insomnia is a symptom of an underlying health problem, such as depression, chronic pain, sleep apnea, or other breathing disorders. But more often than not, insomnia is primarily stress related.

I recommend developing a bedtime ritual that starts with the stretches from Chapter 9 and that may also include wind-down activities such as reading, talking, or breathing exercises such as the ones in Chapter 8. These activities in combination can help calm your mind, relax your muscles, and ease the day's tension — all allowing you to rest more soundly.

Check out the "Stress" section later in this chapter, too.

Low Back Pain

Whether you're sedentary or an elite athlete, tight muscles in your hips, thighs, and buttocks can affect you and actually put so much strain and stress on your lower back that the result is lower back pain. One solution that's been proven to be effective is regular stretching.

Check out Chapter 7 where you'll find a ton of stretches for the hips, thighs, and buttocks, or if you're feeling tightness in your lower back, try the routines in Chapter 6. The entire chapter is dedicated to stretching out your lower back, and I also include a mini back massage that's the best for relieving low back tightness.

Never forget — a healthy back is a strong and flexible back.

Menstrual Cramps

One of the most natural, effective methods of relieving menstrual cramps is to first apply heat from either a warm bath or heating pad and then to engage in some mild stretching. I recommend the stretches I describe in the beginning of Chapter 8. These stretches are very gentle and focus on the pelvic region. If your period causes pain in your lower back, try some of the stretches in Chapter 6 that focus specifically on that area.

Plantar Fasciitis

Plantar fasciitis (plan-tar fash-ee-*ahy*-tis) is an inflammation of a band of fibrous tissue called the *fascia* (fash-ee-*uh*) that runs along the bottom of your foot from the heel to the ball of the foot, which is the *plantar fascia.*

If this area is a problem for you, I recommend stretching the plantar fascia, the *Achilles tendon*, and all the muscles that attach to the Achilles tendon from the calf — the gastrocnemius and the soleus. Check out the lower leg stretches in Chapter 7 for some help.

In the case of chronic irritation of this area, seek your doctor's advice, which most likely may include rest, ice, anti-inflammatory medicine, arch supports, or taping.

Sciatica

Sciatica (sigh-at-i-*kuh*) is pain along the sciatic nerve that's usually caused by a herniated disk of the lumbar region of the spine, and that pain is then radiated to the buttocks and to the back of the thigh. Sometimes sciatica is more broadly defined as pain in the lower back, buttocks, hips, or adjacent parts.

The sciatic nerve travels just under or even sometimes through the piriformis muscle, a small muscle way down deep inside the buttocks that helps the thigh rotate outward. If the piriformis becomes tight, it can irritate or constrict the sciatic nerve, causing symptoms much like actual sciatica.

My favorite piriformis muscle stretch is in Chapter 9 (lying buttocks and hip stretch). It's a heck of a lot cheaper than a visit to the doctor, and it just might do the trick, which means you never had sciatica in the first place. However, if the pain persists for more than four days, you'll have to pay a visit to your doctor after all (and probably shell out some bucks).

Stress

If stress is a constant harsh buzz of daily activity, then think of stretching as a slow, quiet Sunday afternoon you can enjoy any time you like to relieve your stress. The methodical movements in a good flexibility program — like the stretches in Chapter 10 — provide simple, easy activities as you position your body for the next stretch. And then the stretches are followed by periods of quiet stillness as you hold the stretch.

Try concentrating fully on the muscles that you're stretching. This focus helps block out any stray, stress-inducing thoughts. Also, the deep, regular breathing that's so important to effective stretching helps oxygenate your blood, which produces a reduction in overall stress and anxiety.

Tension Headaches

Tension headaches are caused by tight, knotted muscles in your shoulders, neck, scalp, and jaw. These aches tend to occur on both sides of your head and start at the back of your skull and spread forward. The pain is often dull or squeezing, like a tight band or vice. In addition, your shoulders, neck, or jaw may feel tight and sore. To help relieve tension headaches with a series of neck stretches, see Chapter 4.

This tightness is often related to stress, depression, or anxiety, but there can be specific physiological causes as well:

✔ Holding your head in one position for a long time — sitting for an extended period in front of a computer, a microscope, or even a video game

✔ Poor sleep position

✔ Overexerting yourself

✔ Clenching or grinding your teeth

If you tend to get tension headaches, stretching the shoulders and neck helps relax and relieve the tension in your muscles before they cause the headache, and then you can attack the pain before it begins. Stretching won't get your boss off your back, but it can help you stay relaxed whenever he's around.

Chapter 17

Ten Surprising Around-the-House Stretching Accessories

*E*xperts support the fact that stretching before and after physical exercise is important, but it's also extremely helpful to spontaneously stretch throughout the day. Why? Because stretching this and that, here and there, provides several crucial benefits:

- **Energizes you:** When you need an energy boost, and there's no coffee or chocolate in sight, try a stretch or two to get oxygen to your brain. You'll feel great, and you'll skip the calories!

- **Maintains current range of motion:** Even though you're short on time and you missed your stretch class, performing stretches throughout the day helps maintain the range of motion in your joints that you've worked so hard to achieve.

- **Relieves minor aches and pains:** Stretching can relieve the stress and tension created by inactivity or repetitive motion.

So any time can be the right time to stretch when you're at home. And believe it or not your home is full of stretching aids that help you stretch out and feel great. This chapter describes my top-ten stretching props that are commonly found in the average home and instructions on how to use them. Face it: You're surrounded. Now you *really* have no excuse not to stretch!

A Big, Thick Book

Sit on a big book (about the thickness of the average phone book) instead of on the floor when you perform sitting stretches. The book lifts your hips off the floor just enough to take away some of the stress and strain of a tight lower back. And when you don't feel that strain, you can focus more on stretching your hamstrings or inner thighs without rounding your back. Try some of the sitting stretches described in Chapter 7 while sitting on a book, and you should notice how much easier it is to keep your back straight.

After you've gotten proficient at stretching your calves, as described in Chapter 7, you can stand with your heels on the phone book to accentuate the calf stretch.

A Chair

Sitting in a chair too long and too often doesn't loosen and relax your muscles; it *shortens* certain muscles such as your hamstrings, hip flexors, and calves. Nevertheless, a chair can be a very useful and effective stretching prop. I bet you have a chair in just about every room of the house, so as a stretching prop, a chair is extremely accessible. Check out Chapter 10 and Chapter 15 where you use a chair for balance and support with some excellent stretches.

Be careful, especially at work, that the chair you use doesn't have wheels as many computer chairs do. You can use any type of chair as long as it's sturdy and stable.

A Ceiling Beam in Your House or Garage

If you've seen Rocky (and who hasn't?), you know by now that you can hang from an open beam in your house or garage to stretch out your back. At first you may only be able to hold on for a few seconds, but as your grip gets stronger, you'll be able to stay on just long enough to really feel the stretch in your shoulders and back. And every time you do, you'll feel like you're an inch taller.

If you have trouble with this stretch, you may be able to put a chair beneath or beside you to help you "unload."

A Sofa

Although most people think of a couch as primarily being a good place for potatoes to grow roots, believe it or not, your couch can also be a perfect stretching prop because

- ✔ It's comfortable, so it can help you stay relaxed.
- ✔ It's off the floor, so it's not awkward to get into a lot of different positions.
- ✔ You're probably sitting on one right now!

Try the AM/PM stretches I describe in Chapter 9, using the couch instead of the bed.

A Desk

At work it's probably not very professional to put your foot up on your desk, but at home your desk can be an excellent stretching prop.

If you don't have a desk handy, you can do this stretch, using your dining room table or even a hip-high windowsill.

1. **Stand in front of your desk and place your right foot on the edge of the desktop.**

2. **Place your hands on the desk and lean forward so your right knee bends and you feel the stretch in your hamstring/buttocks of your right leg and your hip flexor of your left leg.**

3. **Now step back with your left leg a little from the desk so you can straighten your right leg.**

   Feel a great stretch in the back of your right thigh as you inhale deeply and then exhale.

4. **Repeat the stretch with the left leg.**

A Doorway

I've found that a doorway is a great stretching prop because it's both wonderfully stable and large enough to have many different applications.

Try this shoulder stretch, using your doorway:

1. **Grab onto the molding over the top of the door with your fingertips.**

2. **Bend your knees slightly but keep your feet on the floor until you feel a stretch in your shoulders.**

If you're not tall enough to reach the top of the door, you can use a step stool.

Fireplace Tools

Your fireplace tools don't have to be only decorative anymore; they can actually be great stretching props, too. Using the fireplace tools enhances the effectiveness of the stretch because it adds weight and stability to the movement, allowing you to deepen the stretch, maintain proper posture, and focus on individual muscles.

Try this out:

1. **Pick up either the poker or broom and grab hold of each end with your hands at chest level.**

2. **Twist to the right and left five times each at a slow rhythmic pace to warm up your torso for more vigorous exercise.**

Holding both ends of the poker or broom and then raising it over your head is a great stretch for your shoulders. Add a side bend and you now have a stretch for your waist, too.

A Towel

Although I highly recommend buying a stretching strap to help you with your flexibility program, there's nothing wrong with using the low-cost option of a bath towel or smaller hand towel to help you achieve a comfortable stretch. It doesn't matter whether you're attempting a stretch for the upper or the lower body, using a towel to increase your reach makes the stretch more comfortable. See Chapter 4 or Chapter 7 for a few examples of stretches you can do with a towel.

A Porch Step

Every time you walk into your house with tired feet and tight calves from standing all day or from wearing high heels, you may not realize that you have just walked over the perfect stretching prop to address your aches and pains. Actually, any step is a great place to stretch out your calves, whether on your staircase, your porch, or anywhere else in your house.

Here's how you can use the step to your advantage:

1. **Stand on the step with only the ball of your right foot pressed down as your left foot remains beside it.**

   Make sure that you hold onto a railing or something stable to keep you from falling backwards off the step.

2. **Inhale and as you exhale, slowly lower your heel until you feel a comfortable stretch in your calf.**

3. **Hold the stretch for 10 to 15 seconds.**

   As you breathe, try to gently drop your heel a little lower until you feel a deeper stretch in your calf.

4. **Repeat the stretch on your other leg.**

An excellent variation to help you stretch an even deeper muscle in your calf (the soleus) is to slightly bend the knee of the leg you're stretching. You should feel this variation at the base of your calf.

A Wall

You can use a wall with any stretch that can benefit from firm, stable support. It's smooth and wide, and (I know this sounds a little obvious) adjacent to the floor. It is precisely the fact that a wall is adjacent to the floor that offers you two firm, stable sources of support. For instance, the lying straddle stretch described in Chapter 14 allows you to lie on the floor while your legs are propped up against the wall. This makes the stretch nearly effortless because gravity does all the work.

Index

Notes

BUSINESS, CAREERS & PERSONAL FINANCE

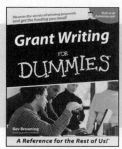

0-7645-5307-0

0-7645-5331-3 *†

Also available:

- Accounting For Dummies †
  0-7645-5314-3
- Business Plans Kit For Dummies †
  0-7645-5365-8
- Cover Letters For Dummies
  0-7645-5224-4
- Frugal Living For Dummies
  0-7645-5403-4
- Leadership For Dummies
  0-7645-5176-0
- Managing For Dummies
  0-7645-1771-6

- Marketing For Dummies
  0-7645-5600-2
- Personal Finance For Dummies *
  0-7645-2590-5
- Project Management For Dummies
  0-7645-5283-X
- Resumes For Dummies †
  0-7645-5471-9
- Selling For Dummies
  0-7645-5363-1
- Small Business Kit For Dummies *†
  0-7645-5093-4

HOME & BUSINESS COMPUTER BASICS

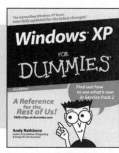

0-7645-4074-2

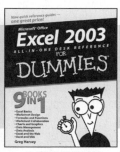

0-7645-3758-X

Also available:

- ACT! 6 For Dummies
  0-7645-2645-6
- iLife '04 All-in-One Desk Reference
  For Dummies
  0-7645-7347-0
- iPAQ For Dummies
  0-7645-6769-1
- Mac OS X Panther Timesaving
  Techniques For Dummies
  0-7645-5812-9
- Macs For Dummies
  0-7645-5656-8
- Microsoft Money 2004 For Dummies
  0-7645-4195-1

- Office 2003 All-in-One Desk Reference
  For Dummies
  0-7645-3883-7
- Outlook 2003 For Dummies
  0-7645-3759-8
- PCs For Dummies
  0-7645-4074-2
- TiVo For Dummies
  0-7645-6923-6
- Upgrading and Fixing PCs For Dummies
  0-7645-1665-5
- Windows XP Timesaving Techniques
  For Dummies
  0-7645-3748-2

FOOD, HOME, GARDEN, HOBBIES, MUSIC & PETS

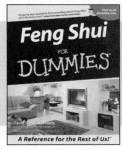

0-7645-5295-3

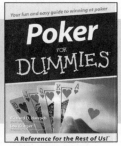

0-7645-5232-5

Also available:

- Bass Guitar For Dummies
  0-7645-2487-9
- Diabetes Cookbook For Dummies
  0-7645-5230-9
- Gardening For Dummies *
  0-7645-5130-2
- Guitar For Dummies
  0-7645-5106-X
- Holiday Decorating For Dummies
  0-7645-2570-0
- Home Improvement All-in-One
  For Dummies
  0-7645-5680-0

- Knitting For Dummies
  0-7645-5395-X
- Piano For Dummies
  0-7645-5105-1
- Puppies For Dummies
  0-7645-5255-4
- Scrapbooking For Dummies
  0-7645-7208-3
- Senior Dogs For Dummies
  0-7645-5818-8
- Singing For Dummies
  0-7645-2475-5
- 30-Minute Meals For Dummies
  0-7645-2589-1

INTERNET & DIGITAL MEDIA

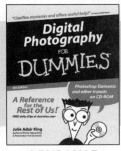

0-7645-1664-7

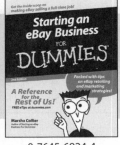

0-7645-6924-4

Also available:

- 2005 Online Shopping Directory
  For Dummies
  0-7645-7495-7
- CD & DVD Recording For Dummies
  0-7645-5956-7
- eBay For Dummies
  0-7645-5654-1
- Fighting Spam For Dummies
  0-7645-5965-6
- Genealogy Online For Dummies
  0-7645-5964-8
- Google For Dummies
  0-7645-4420-9

- Home Recording For Musicians
  For Dummies
  0-7645-1634-5
- The Internet For Dummies
  0-7645-4173-0
- iPod & iTunes For Dummies
  0-7645-7772-7
- Preventing Identity Theft For Dummies
  0-7645-7336-5
- Pro Tools All-in-One Desk Reference
  For Dummies
  0-7645-5714-9
- Roxio Easy Media Creator For Dummies
  0-7645-7131-1

* Separate Canadian edition also available
† Separate U.K. edition also available

Available wherever books are sold. For more information or to order direct: U.S. customers visit www.dummies.com or call 1-877-762-2974.
U.K. customers visit www.wileyeurope.com or call 0800 243407. Canadian customers visit www.wiley.ca or call 1-800-567-4797.

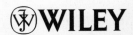 **WILEY**

SPORTS, FITNESS, PARENTING, RELIGION & SPIRITUALITY

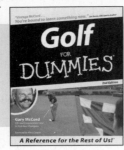

0-7645-5146-9

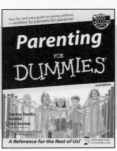

0-7645-5418-2

Also available:
- Adoption For Dummies
  0-7645-5488-3
- Basketball For Dummies
  0-7645-5248-1
- The Bible For Dummies
  0-7645-5296-1
- Buddhism For Dummies
  0-7645-5359-3
- Catholicism For Dummies
  0-7645-5391-7
- Hockey For Dummies
  0-7645-5228-7

- Judaism For Dummies
  0-7645-5299-6
- Martial Arts For Dummies
  0-7645-5358-5
- Pilates For Dummies
  0-7645-5397-6
- Religion For Dummies
  0-7645-5264-3
- Teaching Kids to Read For Dummies
  0-7645-4043-2
- Weight Training For Dummies
  0-7645-5168-X
- Yoga For Dummies
  0-7645-5117-5

TRAVEL

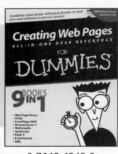

0-7645-5438-7

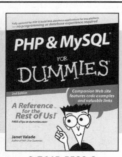

0-7645-5453-0

Also available:
- Alaska For Dummies
  0-7645-1761-9
- Arizona For Dummies
  0-7645-6938-4
- Cancún and the Yucatán For Dummies
  0-7645-2437-2
- Cruise Vacations For Dummies
  0-7645-6941-4
- Europe For Dummies
  0-7645-5456-5
- Ireland For Dummies
  0-7645-5455-7

- Las Vegas For Dummies
  0-7645-5448-4
- London For Dummies
  0-7645-4277-X
- New York City For Dummies
  0-7645-6945-7
- Paris For Dummies
  0-7645-5494-8
- RV Vacations For Dummies
  0-7645-5443-3
- Walt Disney World & Orlando For Dummies
  0-7645-6943-0

GRAPHICS, DESIGN & WEB DEVELOPMENT

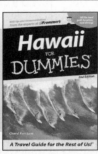

0-7645-4345-8

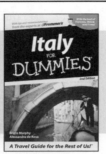

0-7645-5589-8

Also available:
- Adobe Acrobat 6 PDF For Dummies
  0-7645-3760-1
- Building a Web Site For Dummies
  0-7645-7144-3
- Dreamweaver MX 2004 For Dummies
  0-7645-4342-3
- FrontPage 2003 For Dummies
  0-7645-3882-9
- HTML 4 For Dummies
  0-7645-1995-6
- Illustrator CS For Dummies
  0-7645-4084-X

- Macromedia Flash MX 2004 For Dummies
  0-7645-4358-X
- Photoshop 7 All-in-One Desk Reference For Dummies
  0-7645-1667-1
- Photoshop CS Timesaving Techniques For Dummies
  0-7645-6782-9
- PHP 5 For Dummies
  0-7645-4166-8
- PowerPoint 2003 For Dummies
  0-7645-3908-6
- QuarkXPress 6 For Dummies
  0-7645-2593-X

NETWORKING, SECURITY, PROGRAMMING & DATABASES

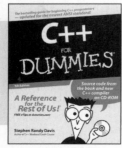

0-7645-6852-3

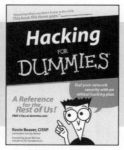

0-7645-5784-X

Also available:
- A+ Certification For Dummies
  0-7645-4187-0
- Access 2003 All-in-One Desk Reference For Dummies
  0-7645-3988-4
- Beginning Programming For Dummies
  0-7645-4997-9
- C For Dummies
  0-7645-7068-4
- Firewalls For Dummies
  0-7645-4048-3
- Home Networking For Dummies
  0-7645-42796

- Network Security For Dummies
  0-7645-1679-5
- Networking For Dummies
  0-7645-1677-9
- TCP/IP For Dummies
  0-7645-1760-0
- VBA For Dummies
  0-7645-3989-2
- Wireless All In-One Desk Reference For Dummies
  0-7645-7496-5
- Wireless Home Networking For Dummies
  0-7645-3910-8